OXFORD MEDICAL PUBLICATIONS

Practical Management of Complex Cancer Pain

D0793160

Oxford Specialist Handbooks published and forthcoming

General Oxford Specialist Handbooks
A Resuscitation Room Guide
Addiction Medicine
Day Case Surgery
Perioperative Medicine, 2e
Pharmaceutical Medicine
Postoperative Complications, 2e
Renal Transplantation

Oxford Specialist Handbooks in Anaesthesia
Anaesthesia for Medical and Surgical Emergencies
Cardiac Anaesthesia
Neuroanaesthesia
Obstetric Anaesthesia
Ophthalmic Anaesthesia
Paediatric Anaesthesia
Regional Anaesthesia, Stimulation and Ultrasound Techniques
Thoracic Anaesthesia

Oxford Specialist Handbooks in Cardiology
Adult Congenital Heart Disease
Cardiac Catheterization and Coronary Intervention
Cardiac Electrophysiology and Catheter Ablation
Cardiovascular Computed Tomography
Cardiovascular Magnetic Resonance
Echocardiography, 2e
Fetal Cardiology
Heart Failure
Hypertension
Inherited Cardiac Disease
Nuclear Cardiology
Pacemakers and ICDs
Pulmonary Hypertension
Valvular Heart Disease

Oxford Specialist Handbooks in Critical Care
Advanced Respiratory Critical Care
Cardiothoracic Critical Care

Oxford Specialist Handbooks in End of Life Care
End of Life Care in Cardiology
End of Life Care in Dementia
End of Life Care in Nephrology
End of Life Care in Respiratory Disease
End of Life in the Intensive Care Unit

Oxford Specialist Handbooks in Neurology
Epilepsy
Parkinson's Disease and Other Movement Disorders
Stroke Medicine

Oxford Specialist Handbooks in Oncology
Practical Management of Complex Cancer Pain

Oxford Specialist Handbooks in Paediatrics
Paediatric Dermatology
Paediatric Endocrinology and Diabetes
Paediatric Gastroenterology, Hepatology, and Nutrition
Paediatric Haematology and Oncology
Paediatric Intensive Care
Paediatric Nephrology, 2e
Paediatric Neurology, 2e
Paediatric Radiology
Paediatric Respiratory Medicine
Paediatric Rheumatology

Oxford Specialist Handbooks in Pain Medicine
Spinal Interventions in Pain Management

Oxford Specialist Handbooks in Psychiatry
Child and Adolescent Psychiatry
Forensic Psychiatry
Old Age Psychiatry

Oxford Specialist Handbooks in Radiology
Interventional Radiology
Musculoskeletal Imaging
Pulmonary Imaging
Thoracic Imaging

Oxford Specialist Handbooks in Surgery
Cardiothoracic Surgery, 2e
Colorectal Surgery
Gastric and Oesophageal Surgery
Hand Surgery
Hepatopancreatobiliary Surgery
Neurosurgery
Operative Surgery, 2e
Oral and Maxillofacial Surgery
Otolaryngology and Head and Neck Surgery
Paediatric Surgery
Plastic and Reconstructive Surgery
Surgical Oncology
Urological Surgery
Vascular Surgery

Oxford Specialist Handbooks in Oncology

Practical Management of Complex Cancer Pain

Edited by

Manohar Sharma

Consultant in Pain Medicine
The Walton Centre
NHS Foundation Trust
Liverpool, UK

Karen H. Simpson

Consultant in Pain Medicine
Leeds Teaching Hospitals
NHS Trust
Leeds, UK

Michael I. Bennett

St Gemma's Professor of Palliative Medicine
Leeds Institute of Health Sciences
University of Leeds
Leeds, UK

Sanjeeva Gupta

Consultant in Pain Medicine
Bradford Royal Infirmary
Bradford, UK

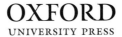

OXFORD
UNIVERSITY PRESS

OXFORD
UNIVERSITY PRESS

Great Clarendon Street, Oxford, OX2 6DP,
United Kingdom

Oxford University Press is a department of the University of Oxford.
It furthers the University's objective of excellence in research, scholarship,
and education by publishing worldwide. Oxford is a registered trade mark of
Oxford University Press in the UK and in certain other countries

© Oxford University Press, 2014

The moral rights of the authors have been asserted

All rights reserved. No part of this publication may be reproduced,
stored in a retrieval system, or transmitted, in any form or by any means,
without the prior permission in writing of Oxford University Press,
or as expressly permitted by law, or under terms agreed with the appropriate
reprographics rights organization. Enquiries concerning reproduction
outside the scope of the above should be sent to the Rights Department,
Oxford University Press, at the address above

You must not circulate this work in any other form
and you must impose this same condition on any acquirer

Published in the United States of America by Oxford University Press
198 Madison Avenue, New York, NY 10016, United States of America

British Library Cataloguing in Publication Data
Data available

Library of Congress Control Number: 2013954328

ISBN 978-0-19-966162-6

Printed in Great Britain by
Ashford Colour Press Ltd, Gosport, Hampshire.

Oxford University Press makes no representation, express or implied, that the drug
dosages in this book are correct. Readers must therefore always check the product
information and clinical procedures with the most up-to-date published product
information and data sheets provided by the manufacturers and the most recent
codes of conduct and safety regulations. The authors and the publishers do not
accept responsibility or legal liability for any errors in the text or for the misuse or
misapplication of material in this work. Except where otherwise stated, drug dosages
and recommendations are for the non-pregnant adult who is not
breast-feeding.

Links to third party websites are provided by Oxford in good faith and
for information only. Oxford disclaims any responsibility for the materials
contained in any third party website referenced in this work.

Preface

Cancer pain management requires the acquisition of appropriate knowledge, skills, and attitudes that support the assessment and management of patients with a variety of causes for cancer pain. The authors assume that readers will have prior education in this field, especially in managing the early stages of cancer pain. This book will be beneficial to doctors and other healthcare professionals working in many disciplines, especially primary care, pain medicine, palliative medicine, oncology, and surgery.

The book focuses on the practical aspects of managing complex cancer pain. This is not a book about theory or the evidence relating to cancer pain management; readers can access that information from current literature and journals. The emphasis is on appropriate collaboration between different specialities.

The book covers pathophysiological aspects of cancer pain, pharmacological therapies, radiotherapy, treating/palliating cancer, as well as managing pain. Interventional pain techniques are covered in detail as these do play a major role in managing some of the more complex pains in these patients. Case histories are presented to give readers insight into the complexities of holistic management, with pain being only one of the factors that distresses patients and families. The book also covers cancer pain management for patients in a community setting. A chapter is devoted to the importance of close collaboration between pain and palliative medicine.

We are pleased that there are contributions from authors with a national and international reputation for expertise in this area. We are grateful to our authors for collecting, editing, and providing some excellent radiographs and figures. It is a privilege to have drawings from Simon Tordoff, whose art work is a legend in the UK pain world. Finally we are grateful to our contributors for their diligence in writing for us and their commitment to excellence and detail. We are also indebted to our publishers for their patience and support.

Manohar Sharma
Karen Simpson
Mike Bennett
Sanjeeva Gupta
2014

Contents

Contributors *ix*

Abbreviations *xi*

Section A Introduction and clinical cases

1 Definition and pathophysiology of complex
  cancer pain   **3**

2 The pharmacological management of cancer pain   **13**

3 Neurolytic blocking agents   **31**

4 The role of surgery in cancer pain management   **41**

5 Oncological management of cancer pain   **53**

6 Pelvic pain   **61**

7 Mesothelioma and chest wall pain   **69**

8 Unilateral upper limb plexopathy pain caused
  by cancer   **79**

9 Diffuse cancer pain in lower half of body   **89**

10 Upper gastrointestinal pain from invasive
   pancreatic cancer   **101**

11 Multiple bone metastasis-related incident pain   **111**

12 Intrathecal pump for cancer pain   **123**

Section B Details of interventional techniques

13 Basic procedure safety and patient considerations
   for cancer pain interventions   **137**

14 Sympathectomy for cancer pain   **147**

15 Vertebroplasty and kyphoplasty in spinal
   metastasis pain   **167**

16 Cervical cordotomy for cancer pain   **181**

17 Intrathecal drug delivery for cancer pain   197

18 Spinal neurolysis   227

19 Trigeminal interventions for head and
   neck cancer pain   239

20 Neurosurgical techniques for cancer pain   251

21 Peripheral nerve blocks including
   neurolytic blocks   263

Section C Collaboration between services

22 Role of collaboration between pain medicine
   and palliative medicine   273

23 Control of complex pain at the end of life
   in hospice or community setting   285

Index 305

Contributors

Professor Michael I. Bennett
St Gemma's Professor of Palliative
Medicine
Leeds Institute of Health Sciences
University of Leeds
Leeds, UK

Dr Stephen Berns
Assistant Professor in Geriatrics
and Palliative Medicine and
Assistant Professor in Internal
Medicine
Mount Sinai, NY, USA

Dr Arun Bhaskar
Consultant in Anaesthesia and Pain
Medicine
The Christie
NHS Foundation Trust
Manchester, UK

Dr Shubhabrata Biswas
Specialist Registrar
Neuroradiology Department
The Walton Centre
NHS Foundation Trust
Liverpool, UK

Dr Kumar S.V. Das
Consultant Neuroradiologist
The Walton Centre
NHS Foundation Trust
Liverpool, UK

Dr Samyadev Datta
Consultant in Pain Medicine
Director, Center for Pain
Management
Hackensack, NJ, USA

Professor Paul Eldridge
Editor in Chief *British Journal of
Neurosurgery* and
Consultant Neurosurgeon
The Walton Centre
NHS Foundation Trust
Liverpool, UK

Dr Chinnamani Eswar
Consultant Clinical Oncologist
Clatterbridge Cancer Centre and
Honorary Lecturer
Liverpool University
Liverpool, UK

Dr Umesh K. Gidwani
Chief, Cardiac Critical Care
Cardiovascular Institute
Mount Sinai School of Medicine
New York, NY, USA

Dr Sanjeeva Gupta
Consultant in Pain Medicine
Bradford Royal Infirmary
Bradford, UK

Dr Heino Hugel
Consultant in Palliative Care
University Hospital Aintree
Liverpool, UK

Dr Subhash Jain
Consultant in Pain Medicine and
Medical Director
Institute of Pain and
Palliative Care
New York, NY, USA

Dr Andrew Jones
Consultant in Anaesthesia and Pain
Medicine
Royal Liverpool University
Hospital
Liverpool, UK

**Dr Dhanalakshmi
Koyyalagunta**
Consultant in Anesthesia and Pain
Medicine
Anderson Cancer Center
Department of Pain Medicine
Houston, TX, USA

Dr Louise Lynch
Consultant in Pain Medicine
Seacroft Hospital
Leeds, UK

Professor Matthew K. Makin
Executive Medical Director
NHS North Wales
Betsi Cadwaladr University
Health Board
Bangor, UK

Dr Kate Marley
Consultant in Palliative Medicine
Warrington and Halton Hospitals
NHS Foundation Trust
Warrington, UK

Dr Manohar Sharma
Consultant in Pain Medicine
The Walton Centre
NHS Foundation Trust
Liverpool, UK

Dr Karen H. Simpson
Consultant in Pain Medicine
Leeds Teaching Hospitals
NHS Trust
Leeds, UK

Dr Devjit Srivastava
Consultant in Anaesthesia and Pain
Medicine
Raigmore Hospital
NHS Highlands
Inverness, UK

Abbreviations

AP	anteroposterior
BITS	bilateral intrathoracic splanchnicectomy
BP	blood pressure
COMT	catechol-O-methyltransferase
CPN	coeliac plexus neurolysis
CSCI	continuous subcutaneous infusion
CSF	cerebrospinal fluid
CT	computed tomography
CYP	cytochrome p450
EBRT	external beam radiation therapy
eGFR	estimated glomerular filtration rate
ERCP	endoscopic retrograde cholangio-pancreatography
GP	general practitioner
ICV	intracerebroventricular
IDDS	intrathecal drug delivery system
IM	intramuscular
IL	interleukin
IR	immediate release
IT	intrathecal
IV	intravenous
ITDD	intrathecal drug delivery
MDT	multidisciplinary team
MR	modified release
MRI	magnetic resonance imaging
NGF	nerve growth factors
NICE	National Institute for Health and Clinical Excellence
NMDA	N-methyl-D-aspartate
NRS	numerical rating scale
NSAID	non-steroidal anti-inflammatory drug
PCA	patient-controlled analgesia
PCC	percutaneous cervical cordotomy
PET	positron emission tomography
PMMA	polymethylmethacrylate
PTM	patient therapy manager
PV	percutaneous vertebroplasty

RF	radiofrequency
RFA	radiofrequency ablation
RVM	rostral ventromedial medulla
SC	subcutaneous
SR	sustained release
SSRI	selective serotonin reuptake inhibitor
TENS	transcutaneous electrical nerve stimulation
TNF	tumour necrosis factor
VAS	visual analogue scale
VRS	verbal rating scale
WFI	water for injection
WHO	World Health Organization

Section A

Introduction and clinical cases

1 Definition and pathophysiology of complex
   cancer pain   3

2 The pharmacological management of
   cancer pain   13

3 Neurolytic blocking agents   31

4 The role of surgery in cancer pain management   41

5 Oncological management of cancer pain   53

6 Pelvic pain   61

7 Mesothelioma and chest wall pain   69

8 Unilateral upper limb plexopathy pain
   caused by cancer   79

9 Diffuse cancer pain in lower half of body   89

10 Upper gastrointestinal pain from invasive
   pancreatic cancer   101

11 Multiple bone metastasis-related incident pain   111

12 Intrathecal pump for cancer pain   123

Definition and pathophysiology of complex cancer pain

Michael I. Bennett

Definition of pain 4
Epidemiology 5
  Prevalence and aetiology 5
  Severity and impact 5
Pathophysiology 7
Complex pain syndromes 8
  Bone pain 8
  Spinal cord compression 8
  Chest wall 8
  Brachial plexopathy 9
  Pancreatic pain 9
  Lumbosacral plexopathy 9
  Pelvic pain 9
Conclusion 10
  Key learning points 10
Further reading 11

Definition of pain

Pain is defined by the International Association for the Study of Pain (IASP) as an 'unpleasant sensory and emotional experience associated with actual or potential tissue damage, or described in terms of such damage'. Chronic pain is defined as 'pain which persists beyond the usual course of healing or is associated with chronic pathological illness which causes continuous pain or pain which recurs at intervals for months or years'.

Pain is always a subjective phenomenon and reflects the patient's own perception of their sensory and emotional experience. As such, it is impossible to quantify directly the sensory and emotional components of one person's pain. The concept of 'total pain' acknowledges the physical, psychological, social, and spiritual influence on a patient's perception of pain and the multidimensional effect it has on a person's life. Good pain control will only be possible if all these aspects are addressed.

Defining the basic mechanisms that sustain pain is often helpful. Nociceptive (or inflammatory) pain is defined as 'pain that arises from actual or threatened damage to non-neural tissue and is due to the activation of nociceptors (pain receptors)'. In contrast, neuropathic pain is defined as 'pain caused by a lesion or disease of the somatosensory nervous system'. It can be further classified as peripheral or central neuropathic pain, and by anatomical site and disease. Both nociceptive and neuropathic are descriptions of pain mechanisms and are not diagnoses. However, from a neurophysiological perspective, many of these mechanisms coexist, suggesting that a rigid distinction between nociceptive and neuropathic is too simplistic. Even in the clinical context, chronic pain usually manifests as a spectrum of nociceptive and neuropathic features; the most useful clinical assessment then becomes whether the pain is *predominantly* neuropathic in nature or not.

Breakthrough pain is the term most widely used to describe variations in quality, intensity, and timing of pain on a background of stable pain control. It can be predictable, unpredictable, spontaneous, or evoked with the same quality or a different quality to the baseline pain.

Pain in a patient with cancer is not synonymous with cancer pain. Cancer pain is strictly pain that results from a direct effect of the cancer, for example, by destruction or compression of soft tissue, bone, or nerves. Pain in a cancer patient may also be caused by cancer treatment or by comorbid disease. For the purposes of this chapter, *complex cancer pain* is defined as cancer pain that is either multifactorial in nature (caused and sustained by a variety of sensory and emotional mechanisms) or is cancer pain that has not responded to simple, conventional treatment approaches. There are examples later in this chapter describing clinical syndromes that are frequently regarded as complex. This is usually because these syndromes do not respond well to conventional treatment, mostly due to the mix of nociceptive and neuropathic pain mechanisms.

Epidemiology

Prevalence and aetiology

Pain occurs in about 50% of patients at diagnosis of cancer and is often the symptom that first alerts patients and their doctors to a problem. Pain is more common as the disease progresses. Systematic reviews have shown that pain occurs in approximately 59% of those on anticancer treatment, 64–74% of those with advanced disease, and in 33% of those that had been cured of their cancer, often caused by cancer treatment. A recent survey of community-based European cancer patients found an overall pain prevalence of 72%. Sites or origins of cancer that are associated with higher prevalence of pain are pancreas, bone, brain, lymphoma, lung, head, and neck. However, the prevalence of pain varies between and within specific cancer diseases, as well as across clinical settings such as hospice, specialist pain clinic, or oncology outpatient services.

As mentioned previously, pain in a patient with cancer may have a variety of causes, many of which coexist. Large observational studies show that in patients with cancer, 76% of pains are caused directly by the cancer, 11% are related to cancer treatment, and around 13% are due to comorbid conditions such as constipation or osteoarthritis. The majority of all pains are nociceptive in nature but around 20% are caused by neuropathic mechanisms. Because cancer patients have around two pains on average, neuropathic pain can affect up to 40% of cancer patients. Although the majority of neuropathic pains are caused by cancer (64%), a significantly higher proportion is caused by cancer treatment (20%) in comparison with all cancer patients. This highlights the growing contribution of cancer treatment to pain in cancer patients, especially that caused by neuropathic mechanisms.

Severity and impact

Observational studies show that at least one-third of patients with cancer rate their pain as either moderate or severe in intensity. In hospitalized patients with cancer, using a 0–10 numerical rating scale, patients reported a pain score of 3.7 for average pain and for two-thirds of patients the severity of their worst pain was rated at greater than 5/10. A large community-based survey found that 93% of those patients who experienced cancer pain at least several times a month rated the severity as moderate to severe, 44% as severe, and 3% regarded it as the worst pain imaginable.

Patients with neuropathic pain have been shown to have greater pain intensity, a worse quality of life, and describe a greater impact on their daily living when compared to patients with nociceptive pain. Similarly those with neuropathic cancer pain have been shown to have a worse quality of life, poorer performance status, use higher doses of opioids, and need a longer time to achieve pain control than those with nociceptive pain. Patients with uncontrolled breakthrough pain are more likely to have a poorer quality of life and be depressed. Psychological distress, defined as anxiety, adjustment disorder, or depression, is also associated with poorer pain outcomes, including greater pain severity and longer duration to reach stable pain control. Significant psychological distress can result in the associated cancer pain being more complex to manage.

The effect of age on cancer pain management is inconsistent. Some studies suggest that no significant differences exist in average pain intensity between younger and older (>75 years of age) cancer patients. However, older people may require less or more analgesia than the younger population, as a result of differences in pharmacokinetics. For example, renal and cognitive impairment (which are more prevalent in older patients) may necessitate dose adjustments or use of alternative medication. Older people may have different attitudes to strong analgesia and therefore be more reluctant to use it.

Pathophysiology

Cancer growth that results in direct tissue damage can induce inflammation. Damage to sensory nerves by infiltration or compression by a cancer can cause neuropathy (painless loss of function) or neuropathic pain. Aside from mechanical damage or distension of sensory nerves, direct stimulation of nociceptors by chemicals released by cancer cells and the accompanying inflammatory mediators also cause pain. These factors include nerve growth factors (NGFs), cytokines such as tumour necrosis factor (TNF), interleukins (such as interleukin (IL)-6), chemokines, prostanoids, and endothelins. These in turn activate receptors on sensory nerves or primary afferent neurons, causing pain. In a recent animal study, anti-NGF therapy almost eliminated pain behaviour in mice with cancer-induced bone pain demonstrating an important role for NGF in this context, and an important new target for pharmacotherapy. Cancer pain is therefore a complex syndrome where inflammatory, neuropathic, and ischaemic mechanisms exist, often at more than one site.

Peripheral sensitization can occur following inflammation which leads to greater activity in sensory neurons. These neurons project onto the spinal cord where they cause more transmitter release, notably substance P, which activates neurokinin-1 (NK1) receptors on central sensory neurons. Spinal neurons also express N-methyl-D-aspartate (NMDA) receptors which activate only with repeated and sustained peripheral input, and which then results in augmentation of peripheral input. This is an important mechanism in central sensitization.

Spinal cord sensory neurons ascend and project to higher brain centres including the thalamus, periaqueductal grey, and the cortex which are involved in the emotional and cognitive perception of pain. These central sensory neurons also connect with the brainstem via the rostral ventromedial medulla (RVM) from which descending, inhibitory neurons project back to the spinal cord which results in damping of peripheral input. These descending mechanisms are also influenced by the limbic system, particularly the thalamus.

Thus the experience of pain is a fine balance between peripheral and central sensitization, modulated by excitatory and inhibitory central mechanisms, and governed by cognitive and emotional influences.

Complex pain syndromes

Bone pain

Bone metastases occur in about 40% of patients with lung, renal, and thyroid cancers, and in about 70% of patients with breast and prostate cancer. Consequently, bone pain is the most common cause of cancer-related pain. It generally presents as a persistent background pain with exacerbations on movement or activity, often called incident or breakthrough pain; these movement-related pains are often difficult to control.

Metastases to vertebral bodies often cause midline pain. Pain from a vertebral pedicle can cause unilateral nerve root pain as can epidural extension of a paravertebral tumour. Disease progression may lead to vertebral body collapse, unilateral or bilateral root pain, and paraplegia or tetraplegia (see following 'Spinal cord compression' section). Thoracic vertebral metastases can result in a band-like pain around the chest wall; if this pain is elicited by coughing, then cord compression is a significant risk. Cervical spine metastases may be associated with Horner's syndrome if significant paravertebral disease exists. Lumbar metastases may be associated with referred pain to the sacroiliac joint or posterior superior iliac crest.

Spinal cord compression

Spinal cord or cauda equina compression affects about 3% of all cancer patients. It is caused by collapse or distortion of a vertebral body or pedicle by metastasis, most often from breast, lung, or prostate cancers. Compression at the lumbar level is commonest (70% of affected patients), followed by thoracic (20%) and cervical (10%). Multiple sites of compression are common.

In the acute stages (initial hours and days), pain is common either at the site of the compression or as a unilateral nerve root pain, associated with distal sensory and motor signs in the legs and pelvis. In more established spinal cord compression, particularly where surgical decompression is not possible, central neuropathic pain also develops because of irreversible spinal cord damage. This can be experienced weeks or some months later as painful dysaesthesias, burning, and sometimes electric shock or shooting pains down the legs.

Chest wall

Infiltration of the chest wall by tumour occurs with primary or metastatic lung cancer, and with mesothelioma. This can result in localized inflammatory pain, often with a pleuritic pattern. If the tumour invades ribs or intercostal nerves, the pain is usually more constant with features of neuropathic pain. In mesothelioma, the first symptom may be a nagging discomfort or mild pain in the chest area or in the back that accompanies breathlessness. As the pleural-based tumour progresses into the chest wall, muscles, and ribs, pain is more severe and is often more diffuse across the whole of the hemithorax. Destruction of sympathetic nerves in the chest wall may also contribute to pain and can lead to unilateral sweating over the chest wall.

Brachial plexopathy

Painful brachial plexopathy in cancer patients may be caused by stretch injury during surgery or invasion from an apical lung cancer (Pancoast's tumour) or metastasis. This pain is often experienced as a burning dysaesthetic pain along the ulnar side of the hand (indicating C7–T1 root involvement) with cramp-like or 'crushing' pains in the forearm. It may be associated with sensory abnormalities in the hand, and Horner's syndrome, an ipsilateral partial ptosis from sympathetic chain involvement.

Pancreatic pain

Pain is not always associated with pancreatic cancer but pain is more likely when the pancreatic ducts are obstructed or pancreatic connective tissue, capillaries, and/or afferent nerves are infiltrated. Pain is especially common and severe when invasion of the coeliac plexus occurs (which can also result from other retroperitoneal or upper gastrointestinal cancers). Pain occurs in about 90% of patients with cancer of the head of the pancreas, particularly if the growth is near the ampulla of Vater. Pain is much less common with cancer of the pancreatic body and tail.

Pancreatic pain usually occurs in the upper abdomen and is usually constant which becomes increasingly severe over a period of time. Pain can also radiate through to the back, between the scapulae, spreading laterally to right and left. Back pain often indicates that retroperitoneal or coeliac plexus infiltration has occurred.

Lumbosacral plexopathy

Lumbosacral plexopathy may be caused by a tumour extending into the intrathecal or epidural spaces, for example, from a retroperitoneal, pelvic floor, or renal bed tumour. Common presentations include pain around the sacrum and in one or both legs with associated weakness that develops later.

Pelvic pain

Cancers of the rectum or colon account for half of all causes of pelvic pain, with cancers of the female reproductive tract accounting for a quarter of cases. Presenting features vary. Central hypogastric pain is common in patients with cancers of the bladder and uterus and is also seen in patients with colorectal cancer, especially if a tumour is invading the bladder or uterus. Unilateral pain in either of the iliac fossae is associated with local recurrence adherent to the lateral pelvic wall.

Rectal tumour and pre-sacral recurrence may cause pain to felt in the perineum or external genitalia, with pain particularly on sitting. This may be mild and described as a feeling of 'pressure', or it may be severe enough to prevent the patient from sitting down. Pre-sacral tumour can lead to lumbosacral plexopathy and pain is experienced around perineum, low back, and, if severe, pain radiates to the upper thighs.

Conclusion

Key learning points
- Cancer pain should be distinguished from pain in a cancer patient—around 25% of pains are caused by cancer treatment or comorbid disease rather than the cancer itself.
- Cancer pain is often a mix of inflammatory and neuropathic mechanisms; the latter are associated with greater use of analgesic medication and poorer quality of life.
- Bone metastases are the most frequent cause of cancer pain, and often quite severe especially if movement-related.

Further reading

Bennett MI, Bagnall AM, Closs SJ (2009). How effective are patient-based educational interventions in the management of cancer pain? Systematic review and meta-analysis. *Pain*, **143**(3), 192–9.

Bennett MI, Rayment C, Hjermstad M, Aass N, Caraceni A, Kaasa S (2012). Prevalence and aetiology of neuropathic pain in cancer patients: a systematic review. *Pain*, **153**, 359–65.

Breivik H, Cherny N, Collett B, de Conno F, Filbet M, Foubert AJ, et al. (2009). Cancer-related pain: a pan-European survey of prevalence, treatment, and patient attitudes. *Ann Oncol*, **20**(8), 1420–33.

Deandrea S, Montanari M, Moja L, Apolone G (2008). Prevalence of under-treatment in cancer pain. A review of published literature. *Ann Oncol*, **19**(12), 1985–91.

Fainsinger RL, Fairchild A, Nekolaichuk C, Lawlor P, Lowe S, Hanson J (2009). Is pain intensity a predictor of the complexity of cancer pain management? *J Clin Oncol*, **27**(4), 585–90.

IASP Task Force on Taxonomy (1994). Part III: Pain terms, a current list with definitions and notes on usage. In Merskey H, Bogduk N (eds) *Classification of Chronic Pain*, 2nd edn, pp. 209–14. Seattle, WA: IASP Press.

The pharmacological management of cancer pain

Matthew K. Makin

Assessment and classification of pain *14*
Principles underpinning effective pain management *16*
Barriers to effective pain management *19*
A systematic approach to prescribing in cancer pain *20*
    Non-opioids *20*
    Weak opioids *20*
    Administration of opioids *21*
Managing adverse effects *23*
    Switching to strong opioid alternatives to morphine *23*
    Oxycodone *23*
    Fentanyl *24*
    Methadone *24*
    Adjuvant and co-analgesics *25*
    Steroids *25*
    Benzodiazepines *26*
    Bisphosphonates *26*
    Anticonvulsants and antidepressants *26*
    Other adjuvants *27*
Conclusion *28*
    Key learning points *28*
Further reading *29*

Assessment and classification of pain

What exactly do we mean by complex or difficult cancer pain? For the patient, and those close to them, pain associated with cancer is never easy, particularly when it is experienced in combination with a constellation of other symptoms leading to debility, distress, loss of function, and an increasing dependence on others. There have been great advances in cancer pain management in many countries and with relatively straightforward interventions the majority of patients should expect good control of symptoms such as pain.

Several forms of cancer pain have been described. Somatic nociceptive pain results from tissue damage and activation of nociceptors that innervate the skin, the ligaments, joints, muscles, and tendons; and is classically well-localized pain. Visceral nociceptive pain is poorly localized and occurs in the hollow organs (often characterized by intermittent colic-type discomfort), in the omentum and mesentery (with a typically large inflammatory component), from organ capsules (e.g. liver), and some other internal organs such as the pancreas. Most patients have a pain syndrome or syndromes that lie on a continuum between nociceptive and neuropathic pain (caused by damage to the peripheral or central nervous system), i.e. there is a mixed aetiology.

Neuropathic pain rarely localizes to the precise point of damage or disruption and patients often describe an area of pain in the distribution of the injured nerve or nerves. Sensation in the area of pain can be unpleasantly abnormal (dysaesthetic) and acutely sensitive—some patients cannot bear to be touched, even by their clothes or bed sheets. The unpleasant sensations characteristic of neuropathic pain are often associated with particular descriptive terms, some that patients commonly use include intense aching, shooting, and tingling. Several scales such as the Leeds Assessment of Neuropathic Symptoms and Signs (LANSS) have been specifically developed to evaluate various symptoms associated with neuropathic pain and can play a useful role in objective assessment.

Pain can be directly related to the cancer or due to infiltration or compression of the peripheral or central nervous system or through the development of painful paraneoplastic neuropathy. Cancer treatment is also a common cause of neuropathic pain and can arise from complications of surgery (thoracotomy and pain following head and neck or groin dissection), and also through chemotherapy-induced peripheral neuropathy (particularly with platinum-containing compounds, vinca alkaloids, and drugs like bortezomib and lenalidomide).

To manage cancer pain successfully, early and methodical assessment is essential. This assessment should take into account all the available information: the history of the pain, its physical effects and manifestations, the functional limitations the pain forces on the individual, and in particular the temporal variation and subjective descriptors as well as objective measures of severity. Visual analogue scales (VASs), numerical and verbal rating scales (NRSs, VRSs) can help with this objective assessment and the McGill Pain Questionnaire and the Brief Pain Inventory are multidimensional tools, incorporating NRSs and VRSs that have been validated in a number of cultures and countries.

A thorough clinical history is important with particular attention paid to the temporal nature of the cancer pain syndrome. This will characterize whether there is a background pain of constant or variable intensity, and if there is episodic or 'breakthrough' pain that has been defined as 'a transient exacerbation of pain that occurs either spontaneously, or in relation to a specific predictable or unpredictable trigger, despite relatively stable and adequately controlled background pain'. If patients have episodic pain it is also helpful to identify whether it is spontaneous or predictably evoked by movement or coughing. The clinical history will influence the choice of the appropriate treatment strategy. In pain that is predominantly episodic in nature the use of escalating doses of modified-release strong opioid analgesia can lead to the patient becoming sedated or experiencing unwanted, or unpleasant adverse effects, whereas strategies that either prevent the trigger to the pain episode, or manage, or pre-empt the pain with short-acting analgesia can lead to a better balance between side effects and analgesia.

The patient must also have a systematic clinical examination in order to reach a reliable diagnosis, with particular attention to sensory testing. Reference to appropriate plain film, isotope bone scan, or cross-sectional imaging (with computed tomography (CT), magnetic resonance imaging (MRI)), all help support the clinical diagnosis of the pain syndrome or syndromes. In some cases positron emission tomography (PET) is necessary to characterize the pathology of the pain syndrome when all clinical suspicion points to a malignant origin. The correct diagnosis of the pain syndrome is necessary in order to avoid unnecessary or ineffective prescribing.

Principles underpinning effective pain management

When managing pain, complex or otherwise associated with cancer, the challenge for us as clinicians is to find an appropriate balance between pain relief and the unintended or side effects of our intervention. The primary objective should be, rather than necessarily an expectation of abolishing pain completely, aiming to consign it to the background; turning the volume of any pain down so the patient can sleep, rest, and function when they choose.

The palliation of pain requires the clinician to appreciate the factors particular to the individual: their prognosis; whether comorbidity such as renal or hepatic failure are present; the patient's exposure to previous treatment and their experiences, and their fears or concerns about certain medication; the potential for drug interactions; and their willingness to accept any potential side effects of medication. Some patients may not even report pain for a variety of reasons—whether due to fear, concern about financial implications, or as a result of religious or cultural influences. This emphasizes the role of the clinician not only as a skilled prescriber, but someone who is an accomplished listener; able to demonstrate an empathetic approach and offer compassionate care.

The principle of 'first do no harm' that underpins the practice of medicine is never more important than in the face of advanced or life-limiting disease; avoiding 'wasted' days suffering distressing side effects such as delirium, excessive or unwanted sedation, or hallucinations and constipation are just as important as achieving rapid and effective pain relief. Side effects should be therefore monitored, and mitigated for; prescription of a regular laxative, for example, is necessary in the majority of cases. What is required is a 'bespoke', rather than an 'off-the-peg' approach to the patient's analgesic regimen; that needs time and industry during the first assessment, and will require altering and carefully tailoring the combination of drugs to the individual.

The success of this approach is dependent on several things: firstly, the accuracy of the clinical assessment and in particular the diagnosis of the pathology causing the pain syndrome/s; secondly, a systematic and rational approach to analgesic interventions that are familiar to the patient, clinician, and the team supporting and caring for the patient (including when and how to take regular medication and what to do in the event of breakthrough and other episodic pains); and thirdly, repeated evaluations at appropriate intervals, with judicious alterations of dose and choice of analgesic and the management of any unpleasant or unwanted side effects.

These three principles put the patient's welfare at the heart of treatment, and indeed where possible the patient should be the clinicians' closest partner, with agreed goals of treatment, shared information about drug and non-drug options, and opportunities for routine, and, where necessary, rapid reassessment, information, or advice being available.

The clinician is therefore advised to use a patient-centred, holistic, and multimodal approach to cancer pain management, combining both the science and the art of medicine. This is not simply a pragmatic approach but one that respects the complex pharmaco-genetics and genomics that mean that individuals can behave differently and in some cases unpredictably to drug therapy.

Drug treatment will play a role in pain management in the majority of cases of cancer pain, and the principles of the World Health Organization (WHO) analgesic ladder should be applied; with judicious use of regular non-opioids and appropriate adjuvant analgesics, this enables patients to use lower doses of opioid analgesia than if opioids were used as mono-therapy alone. Oral morphine is the typical opioid of first choice, although in some cases, to achieve a satisfactory balance between side effects and analgesia, it may be necessary to either switch to an alternative opioid, or an alternative route of administration

The case of this young mother illustrates the importance of treating each patient as an individual:

'Patient A was a 42-year-old patient who had lived for many years with advanced breast cancer; in her final months the disease had more recently progressed insidiously and become resistant to chemotherapy. Painful cutaneous deposits developed over the anterior chest wall and she developed a painful neuropathy due to brachial plexus infiltration; despite this she was reticent to escalate her analgesic regime that consisted of modified-release morphine 30mg twice a day, paracetamol 1g four times a day, and gabapentin 300mg once only at night. A single parent, she had a 5-year-old daughter and did not want to be too sedated during the night through concern she might not hear her daughter if she woke. If she had particularly troublesome episodic pain during the day, she would call her mother to sit with her daughter, take 10–20mg of immediate-release morphine, and rest in bed for an hour or two. This approach suited her and her family; she titrated the analgesia herself and died peacefully at home. In her final days, and when she was too weak to swallow, medication (morphine 40mg, and clonazepam 1mg) was given via a continuous subcutaneous infusion (CSCI). This was possible only through the support of the community nursing team, who had the facility to ring for specialist advice if required.'

In short, pain associated with cancer should not be considered as a condition of analgesic deficiency, rather symptoms should be identified as being either directly or indirectly associated with the cancer, a complication or consequence of the treatment of the cancer, or a separate, or even pre-existing comorbidity. These symptoms should be assessed for their severity and impact upon the patient's ability to function and should be managed using a combination of disease-modifying treatments, non-drug and lifestyle approaches, as well as pharmacotherapy and, when necessary, interventional analgesia. Gaps in the existing evidence-based literature mean that the art of practice in this setting is skilfully integrating pain management approaches with the control of other symptoms.

Accurate identification of the pathology underlying the pain syndrome also enables timely intervention with either regional analgesia or interventional neuroablative procedures.

Taking into account the patient's performance status, prognosis, and preferences is essential to selecting the most appropriate strategy: a patient with a poor performance status with a very limited prognosis may not survive long enough to benefit from a surgical or oncological approach to pain management; equally it cannot be assumed that such patients would naturally accept the sedative effects of escalation or addition of centrally active analgesics. Other patients near to the end of life might welcome the opportunity to rest or doze more, particularly if symptoms have disturbed sleep patterns, and therefore may more readily accept the sedative effects of opioid or adjuvant analgesia; or medication with anxiolytic or sedative intent. In saying this, however, there is no evidence that appropriate use of opioid analgesia in the last days of life hastens death—although this is a popular misconception.

A negotiation is necessary with each individual patient and, with their consent, their family—making an assumption they have capacity to take part in balanced decision-making unless proven otherwise, and in cases where the patient is unable to do so, decisions should be made by the primary prescriber based upon the principle of maximizing overall benefit for the patient.

Barriers to effective pain management

The extent of the disease or tissue damage is also not directly associated with the patient's perception and their response to the pain; and must be seen in the context of their individual experience of suffering. There is a need therefore for the treating clinician as far as possible to connect and empathize with the patient, their individual circumstances, and the nature of their suffering. Suffering has been defined as:

'A state of severe distress associated with events that threaten the intactness of the person, occurring when an impending destruction of the person is perceived; it continues until the threat of disintegration has passed or until the integrity of the person can be restored in some other manner.'

An appreciation of some of these psycho-social, existential and spiritual issues, engaging appropriate health, social care and other support workers should happen with an approach of active pain management. It should be acknowledged that failure to manage depression and anxiety adequately is one reason that pain management can appear complex or challenging.

Communication between teams is important; and central to this (and in order to avoid incoherent polypharmacy) is the identification of who the primary prescriber is. Most pain management can occur in primary care and community with only a small percentage of patients requiring specialist pain management. So the patient's family doctor, or indeed their oncologist during active treatment may fulfil the role of 'primary prescriber', (and indeed a response to primary anti-cancer therapy, in terms of chemo-, biological, hormone or radiotherapy may be the single most important and effective analgesic intervention). In a small number of cases it is necessary for the palliative care physician, or pain specialist, to not only advise, but to function as the primary prescriber.

When exploring beliefs and worries about analgesia patients should also be given an opportunity to express their concerns about either starting new analgesic drugs or dose adjustments. Some patients have a natural aversion to taking regular medication; others may hold the misconception that if drugs are used to manage pain at an early stage there will be 'nothing left' if pain escalates at the later or terminal stages of the disease. Other patients may have fears of addiction, or become distressed by the perceived implications that starting opioid drugs, particularly morphine, have on their prognosis. Many clinicians are fearful that respiratory depression is a risk when prescribing strong opioids in cancer pain; however, this is rarely clinically relevant in chronic therapy as tolerance builds quickly.

So, choice of pharmacological therapy will be dependent on a number of complex and correlated factors. Some relatively straightforward principles can be applied though; analgesics given regularly, in combination, by mouth, with regular assessment, and escalation or de-escalation of pain informing whether a step up or a step down the ladder is appropriate.

A systematic approach to prescribing in cancer pain

Non-opioids

In the first instance regular non-opioid analgesics such as paracetamol can be an effective first step; used regularly via the oral route it is well tolerated, has no centrally acting side effects, and is unlikely to interact with any of the patient's other medication. In the hospital setting paracetamol can also be administered intravenously. Non-steroidal anti-inflammatory drugs (NSAIDs such as diclofenac, ibuprofen) can be used for inflammatory pain associated with bone pain, or the visceral pain associated with peritoneal metastases. Diclofenac given via the rectal route is useful when the oral route is not possible, or when patients experience ligamentous aches and pains associated with prolonged periods of immobility in bed in the final weeks or days of life. Ketoprofen crosses the blood–brain barrier and so may offer particular utility in patients with headache secondary to cerebral primary or secondary tumours; as may Ketorolac given via CSCI in patients with uncontrolled pain where there is a significant inflammatory component, e.g. patients with widespread bone metastases. The regular use of NSAIDs risks pathological toxicity developing; most notably acute kidney injury, gastric ulceration, and because of antiplatelet effects, bleeding and/or haemorrhage. Interactions with other drugs should be carefully considered; the most significant risk being with warfarin.

Opioids, unlike NSAIDs, cause pharmacological rather than pathological toxicity, i.e. their unwanted effects are not associated with tissue damage *per se*, rather during chronic use, either predictable dose-related side effects (e.g. constipation and sedation) or less predictable effects (that have been referred to as opioid-induced neurotoxicity), e.g. myoclonus, hallucinations, and delirium.

Weak opioids

Codeine is typically the 'weak opioid' of first choice, often given regularly at doses of 16mg or 60mg via the oral route in combination with 1g of paracetamol four times a day. Codeine is a naturally occurring alkaloid in opium, however, as a pro-drug, its analgesic properties only arise following conversion in the liver to morphine and its other metabolite codeine-6-glucoronide; processes catalysed by the cytochrome p450 (CYP) enzyme CYP2D6, and the metabolic isoenzyme uridine diphosphate glucuronosyl transferase UGT2B7 respectively. Genetic variation of CYP2D6 can lead to particular phenotypes ranging from the poor metabolizer with two non-functioning alleles (representing up to 10% of the general population and with patients typically showing a poor analgesic response to codeine) to the extensive or ultra-rapid metabolizer with duplicate or multiple genes (representing up to 2% of the population, metabolizing the drug more quickly than other patients). Notable drug interactions are with dexamethasone that enhances metabolism through enzyme induction and with selective serotonin reuptake inhibitors (SSRIs) that reduce or stop conversion by enzyme inhibition. Although dihydrocodeine is another drug classed as a 'weak opioid' it is not used widely via the oral route in the palliative care setting; although in cases of drug-resistant headache caused by intracerebral malignancy, it has been reported as being effective given as a CSCI at doses ranging from 100–200mg over 24 hours. In some cases clinicians choose to omit the second step of the WHO analgesic ladder in order to achieve prompt pain relief; however, it must be recognized there are risks of toxicity, losing the confidence of the patient if titration is carried out too rapidly.

Administration of opioids

When patients have escalating pain, or pain that is not controlled to the patient's satisfaction despite regular non-opioids and weak opioids, the dilemma for the clinician is whether to add an adjuvant analgesic or to take a step up the ladder and prescribe a strong opioid regularly. Morphine is still the strong opioid of first choice in the management of chronic cancer pain, and most healthcare professionals in primary and secondary care are familiar with its use. In general it is made available to patients in two oral formulations: modified (MR) and immediate release (IR) and can, when necessary be administered by subcutaneous (SC) injection and CSCI.

Most clinicians would start a patient on a typical dose of between 10mg and 20mg of MR morphine twice a day, with IR morphine at an initial dose of 2.5–5mg being available initially to manage episodic or breakthrough pain. Higher doses may be chosen in patients established on long-term weak opioids; and lower doses are preferred in cases of frailty and associated comorbidity such as renal impairment. Indeed in patients with severe renal impairment (estimated glomerular filtration rate (eGFR) <30mL/min) MR morphine should be avoided if possible, and if the patient requires an opioid, an alternative such as fentanyl, alfentanil, or methadone should be considered.

Traditional teaching has been to initiate oral morphine by titrating the regular dose of oral IR morphine given every 4 hours, however a study has confirmed that titrating with the regular dose of oral MR morphine given every 12 hours (with IR morphine given as a 'rescue' analgesia) has been proven to be just as effective and safe.

As yet, no other drug has shown sufficient advantages to supersede oral morphine as the strong opioid of first choice in chronic cancer pain; systematic reviews and comparative trials with other opioids such as oxycodone, fentanyl, hydromorphone, and methadone have confirmed no evidence that these other alternative opioids demonstrate superiority (a clinical trial comparing regular methadone with morphine was halted due to excess morbidity and mortality in the methadone group). Morphine is not expensive, and indeed its various preparations, morphine MR and IR are significantly cheaper than other strong opioids such as oxycodone and the newer transdermal, buccal, sublingual, and intranasal formulations of other strong opioids such as fentanyl or buprenorphine.

A systematic review of the effectiveness of oral morphine, examined 54 studies showing that morphine gives good relief for cancer pain and is effective in a wide dose-range when administered by mouth. There is no ceiling dose per se; and dose increments are made by increasing the dose of MR 'regular' and IR 'rescue' medication by 30–50%. With the appropriate use of non-opioid and adjuvant analgesia the majority of patients require

<200mg morphine over 24 hours; however, the genetic variations between patients mean that there are unique differences in response to morphine. This can be the result of differences in pharmacokinetics (in metabolism and transport of morphine) or in pharmacodynamics (in interaction with genetic variants of the opioid receptor or intracellular signalling systems).

Oral absorption can range from 20–80% between patients, and some genetic mutations mean that the transport protein P-glycoprotein that helps the opioid cross cell membranes does not function effectively; this leads to either too little or too much cellular transport of morphine. Genetic variation of the catechol-O-methyltransferase (COMT) gene has also been shown to significantly affect efficacy of morphine in cancer pain treatment as well. COMT is an enzyme important in the modulation of pain because of its role (amongst other things) in the degradation of dopamine, adrenaline, and noradrenaline.

Managing adverse effects

Like any other centrally acting drug morphine has side effects. With chronic therapy the spectrum of these can range from nausea, constipation, and mild cognitive impairment to dose-limiting somnolence and, in some cases, myoclonus and hallucinations. Tolerance to respiratory depression develops rapidly, allowing morphine to be used in chronic cancer pain without significant respiratory risk. Constipation is an inevitable side effect (as it is with codeine) mediated via enteric as well as spinal and possibly supraspinal opioid receptors. Significant tolerance to this side effect does not appear to develop, necessitating the use of regular laxatives with few exceptions.

In most cases the cognitive impairment and dizziness that occurs within a few days of commencing therapy or dose escalation is self-limiting. Morphine may be associated with toxicity in patients with renal impairment due to accumulation of the active metabolites morphine-3-glucoronide and morphine-6-glucoronide. A strong opioid alternative to morphine is necessary in some cases; however, before doing this, measures such as dose reduction, appropriate rehydration, and the use of adjuvant medication to manage side effects (such as antiemetics, or small doses of haloperidol 0.5mg at night to manage vivid dreams) should be considered.

Switching to strong opioid alternatives to morphine

Alternatives to morphine have a role if patients develop intolerable neurotoxicity during continuous use (e.g. agitation, delirium, myoclonic jerks, hallucinations, hyperalgesia, or allodynia), and are unresponsive to simple measures such as dose reduction, or when dose reduction leads to increased pain.

Another indication is when the dose-limiting side effects of morphine prohibit dose escalation leading to inadequate pain relief (despite use of co-analgesics and techniques appropriate to the pain syndrome).

In patients with malabsorption, dysphagia or when compliance is poor, substitution to a transdermal patch such as fentanyl or buprenorphine is reasonable to consider but only if analgesic requirements are stable. If pain is unstable a CSCI of diamorphine/morphine (or in cases of severe renal impairment) alfentanil should be used in preference.

Oxycodone

Oxycodone also has an important role as a second-line alternative to oral morphine. It is available in MR and IR preparations, and therefore can be carefully titrated in the event of an unstable or escalating pain syndrome. As it is available as an injectable it can also be given as an intermittent infusion or CSCI. In a recent study that compared oxycodone head to head with morphine (with the option of switching from one to the other if dose-limiting side effects to the first opioid resulted in inadequate analgesia) although oxycodone did not demonstrate sufficiently significant advantages to suggest it should be used in preference to morphine first line, the majority of cancer patients in the study achieved good pain control given the ability to switch opioids if indicated.

Fentanyl

Fentanyl is a potent synthetic (roughly 75× more potent than oral morphine) opioid with a low molecular weight and good lipid solubility that can be administered via a transdermal patch. It has some clinical advantages over oral morphine, a reduced incidence of constipation, and metabolites that do not accumulate in renal failure. It is useful if the oral route is unreliable—particularly if absorption and/or compliance are problematic. Some patients may prefer to use transdermal fentanyl because of the convenience of changing a patch every 72 hours rather than taking medication orally every 12 hours. Transdermal fentanyl offers less utility, however, when managing pain that is episodic, unstable, or escalating; titration is difficult, as many clinicians find it hard to decide when, or whether, to increase the dose of the patch, or the time interval between dose increments. Rapid and injudicious dose escalation in these circumstances risks the development of toxicity.

Methadone

In many of the discussion forums on pain management and palliative medicine methadone is suggested as the answer to a variety of 'challenging' pain syndromes. Methadone can be a useful alternative to other strong opioids, but its use should not be considered lightly. Methadone is a synthetic strong opioid analgesic. It is cheap and is the only long-acting opioid that can be given as a liquid. It is well known for its utility in the treatment of opioid dependence.

The use of methadone in the treatment of pain was, until recently, limited to a few individuals working from specialist centres. However, over the past decade anecdotal reports and a number of open case series and clinical trials have described the successful use of methadone, principally in cancer pain syndromes that have responded poorly to high doses of other strong opioids.

Methadone does not accumulate in renal failure nor does it cross renal dialysis membranes, rather the majority (about 70%) is excreted via the gut. These properties suggest advantages over other strong opioids in patients with renal impairment or on dialysis because of end-stage renal failure.

Methadone is characterized by a large inter-individual variation in pharmacokinetics that may cause accumulation if doses are too large or the dosing intervals are too short over a long period of time. This is the main reason why attention is required when using this drug for the treatment of chronic cancer pain. Methadone has the potential to control pain that does not respond to morphine or other opioids, because methadone shows incomplete cross-tolerance with other mu-opioid receptor agonist analgesics.

There have been many case reports of the successful use of methadone in cancer pain as well as an increasing number of retrospective and prospective open case studies. The primary indication for considering methadone as an alternative strong opioid is when a patient with a challenging pain syndrome develops resistant dose-limiting side effects to morphine or other strong opioids, usually with relatively high doses, e.g. mean equivalent daily dose (MEDD) of morphine >200mg. These side effects will often prohibit escalation of the previous opioid dose and give rise to inadequate analgesia, despite the use of adjuvant analgesics and/or techniques appropriate to the pain syndrome. In such circumstances methadone may have specific advantages as an alternative strong opioid because of the synergistic actions of its opioid and non-opioid effects, lack of active metabolites, and the unidirectional cross tolerance it displays with other mu-opioid agonists. In a double blind randomized controlled trial methadone showed an analgesic advantage over placebo in patients with treatment-resistant neuropathic pain, and has demonstrated analgesic activity in other neuropathic pain syndromes.

There is no evidence that methadone is superior to morphine as an analgesic. It is not easy to switch and several approaches have been recommended to switch safely to methadone from the previous opioid. Because of the unidirectional cross tolerance associated with methadone there is no agreed approach of converting from methadone to other opioids. It can be hazardous because of its pharmacology; it is best initiated therefore as an alternative opioid in a specialist inpatient setting by a team experienced in its use. It is, however, cheap and anecdotal experience suggests it may be useful in challenging pain syndromes where patients have failed to tolerate adequate doses of alternative opioids.

Adjuvant and co-analgesics

At every step of the WHO analgesic ladder there is the option of using adjuvant or co-analgesic medication. These are drugs such as anticonvulsants (gabapentin, clonazepam) or antidepressants (amitriptyline, duloxetine) whose primary use is other than as an analgesic. Corticosteroids such as dexamethasone have particular utility and can be given orally or subcutaneously in the palliative care setting. Dexamethasone appears to be particularly effective in severely painful neuropathies due to nerve compression or infiltration by tumour, hepatic capsular stretch pain, headache associated with cerebral oedema due to malignancy, or other inflammatory mediated pain such as peritoneal or multiple bone metastases.

Steroids

Steroids such as dexamethasone should be used with great caution as in the short term mood disorder, insomnia, and hyperglycaemia can occur, and in the longer term, adrenal insufficiency, disabling proximal myopathy, compromise of skin integrity, and risk of infection due to their immunosuppressant effect can complicate treatment. The approach many clinicians use is to offer steroids as a 'pulse' of therapy given for a 5-day trial of treatment. If the patient was not previously on steroids the drug can be stopped after 5 days (if ineffective), or titrated down gradually every 3–5 days until the lowest effective dose is reached. As such, dexamethasone as an adjuvant analgesic is best suited for use in patients with a limited prognosis, and because of the inherent risks the 'primary prescriber' should take responsibility for the dose and duration of treatment. This is particularly important now that the response of too many of the new molecular targeted agents used to combat cancer (e.g. ipilimumab in melanoma) requires an unsuppressed immune system.

Benzodiazepines

Muscle spasms, myofascial pains, and ligamentous aches and pains related to cancer (or immobility as performance status deteriorates) can be helped by drugs such as diazepam, clonazepam, and baclofen in addition to careful nursing. Although similar in efficacy to baclofen, diazepam and clonazepam are associated with more daytime drowsiness.

Bisphosphonates

Bisphosphonate drugs such as zoledronic acid can offer utility as an adjuvant to treat bone pain as a consequence of hormone-relapsed prostate cancer (where localized surgery or radiotherapy is either not indicated or not possible); but there is insufficient evidence to support their routine use in other cancers to manage pain associated with bone metastases, and they are often reserved for cases that respond poorly to regular analgesics.

Although generally well tolerated, bisphosphonates can cause myalgia, and carry the risk of deterioration in renal function, as well as the more recently identified complication of osteonecrosis of the jaw. Bone is involved in about 75% of cases of metastases and pain can be difficult to treat because of the combination of background, spontaneous, and episodic movement-related pain. Whilst opioids and non-opioids can be effective in managing the background pain, the spontaneous and episodic pains can be more challenging, and preclinical studies suggest a role for drugs such as gabapentin. The human monoclonal antibody denosumab has also shown improved pain prevention and comparable pain palliation to zoledronic acid in patients with advanced breast cancer and bone metastases.

Anticonvulsants and antidepressants

Damage, or dysfunction, of the central or peripheral nervous system may cause neuropathic pain in cancer patients and is present in about 50% of patients who have pain that is difficult to control. Gabapentin, a drug that was originally developed for the treatment of epilepsy, is one of many drugs that can be used as adjuvant in the management of many cancer-related neuropathic pain syndromes. Other drugs such as clonazepam (which has the advantage of being able to be given via CSCI), or the antidepressants amitriptyline and duloxetine have shown benefit in neuropathic pain syndromes. All these centrally acting medications should be used cautiously and judiciously, with regular periods of reassessment.

Treatment choices in this setting are often guided by evidence generated by studies examining non-malignant neuropathic pain, the first-choice adjuvant is not always effective, however, sequential trials can be time consuming and risk exposing the patient to unwanted adverse effects. This is particularly true of the more novel co-analgesics, which may have shown a potential benefit in the laboratory, or anecdotal success in small numbers of patients. There is an understandable temptation to extrapolate results from basic science and non-cancer pain, directly to cancer patients.

A balance is required, between the insouciant employment of unproven therapies and a reluctance to only use agents that have shown unequivocal effectiveness in double-blinded controlled trials.

The successful use of adjuvants in this setting therefore depends on the primary prescriber's familiarity with the co-analgesic in question and the application of this knowledge to the individual patient and their circumstances. Careful dose titration and regular reassessment is crucial, as improvement of quality of life is the primary goal, so avoidance of unpleasant or unwanted side effects should be the main concern. Tricyclic antidepressants such as amitriptyline (because of their anticholinergic effects) should be used with caution in elderly or very frail patients at risk of delirium, and as gabapentin is entirely excreted by the renal system it should be prescribed carefully to patients with impaired kidney function with a reduction in total daily dose and a wider dose administration schedule (i.e. from three times a day dose schedules, to either twice or once a day).

Other adjuvants

The same principle of caution should apply to other adjuvants such as the anticonvulsants sodium valproate, lamotrigine and clonazepam as well as membrane stabilizers such as mexiletine, and antidepressants such as venlafaxine and duloxetine. All these drugs have shown they can have a role as co-analgesics but as they act centrally none are without their side effects and should therefore be used watchfully as part of a multimodal approach to pain management. This approach can utilize topical agents such as menthol, capsaicin, and lidocaine that avoid the risk of central side effects, particularly in frail and elderly patients. The 5% lidocaine patch can be a useful intervention in some patients who have dysaesthetic pain and allodynia in a circumscribed area, and studies are currently evaluating the safety and effectiveness of topical clonidine.

When the oral route is not possible, and in the last days of life if patients are too weak to safely take their adjuvant analgesics, clonazepam can be given as a CSCI at a dose of 1–3mg over 24 hours, as can the NMDA receptor antagonist ketamine, which can also be used earlier in cases of severe neuropathic pain. There has been much interest in the use of NMDA receptor antagonists in the management of neuropathic pain. Ketamine, dextromethorphan, and the strong opioid methadone have been suggested as having putative action at the NMDA receptor. Non-competitive antagonists at this receptor complex have been shown, in animal models, to block the hypersensitivity seen in neuropathic pain, potentiating the analgesic action and attenuating the development of tolerance to morphine that is seen in the 'wind up' that is typical of neuropathic pain states. This marked synergy between NMDA receptor antagonists and opioid agonists has been described with the administration of ketamine via CSCI for the treatment of intractable cancer pain. Starting doses of 50–100mg via CSCI over 24 hours are typically used, doses can be adjusted by 50mg every 24 hours to a maximum of 600mg over 24 hours. Most clinicians will also use small doses of either haloperidol or midazolam to attenuate any dysphoric side effects. The use of ketamine as an adjuvant in combination with opioids will necessitate an opioid dose reduction of 30–50%.

Conclusion

Key learning points

- A pathological diagnosis of the pain syndrome is necessary to inform appropriate treatment strategies.
- A holistic assessment should include an appreciation of subjective components of 'suffering' as well as objective measures of pain.
- Objectives of treatment should be negotiated and regularly reassessed with the patient, and those close to them.
- Patients and those close to them should have access to information about drug and non-drug interventions for pain and have appropriate access to advice and support.
- Analgesic choice should be rational and systematic with close attention to the risks and management of unwanted side effects.

Further reading

Buga S, Sarria J (2012). The management of pain in metastatic bone disease. *Cancer Control*, **19**(2), 154–66.

Cassell EJ (1982). The nature of suffering and the goals of medicine. *N Engl J Med*, **306**(11), 639–45.

Cleeland CS, Body JJ, Stopeck A, von Moos R, Fallowfield L, Mathias SD, et al. (2013). Pain outcomes in patients with advanced breast cancer and bone metastases: results from a randomized, double-blind study of denosumab and zoledronic acid. *Cancer*, **119**(4), 832–8.

Colvin L, Forbes K, Fallon M (2006). Difficult pain: an ABC of palliative care. *BMJ*, **332**(6), 1081–3.

Davies AN, Dickman A, Reid C, Stevens AM, Zeppetella G (2009). The management of cancer-related breakthrough pain: recommendations of a task group of the Science Committee of the Association for Palliative Medicine of Great Britain and Ireland. *Eur J Pain*, **13**, 331–8.

Rakvåg T, Ross J, Sato H, Skorpen F, Kaasa S, Klepstad P (2008). Genetic variation in the catechol-o-methyltransferase (COMT) gene and morphine requirements in cancer patients with pain. *Mol Pain*, 4, 64. Available at: <http://www.molecularpain.com/content/pdf/1744-8069-4-64.pdf> (accessed 20 April 2013).

Riley J, Bradford R, Droney J, Gretton S, Sato H, Kennett A, et al. (2012). *A randomized controlled trial comparing response to first line opioid and clinical efficacy of opioid switching*. Presented as abstract/poster at European Association of Palliative Care Meeting 2012.

Ripamonti C (2012). Pain management. *Ann Oncol*, **23**(10), 294–301.

Walker PW, Palla S, Be-Lian P, Kaur G, Zhang K, et al. (2008). Switching from methadone to a different opioid: what is the equianalgesic dose ratio? *J Palliat Med*, **11**(8), 1103–8.

Wiffen PJ, McQuay HJ (2010). Oral morphine for cancer pain. *Online Cochrane Summaries*. Available at: <http://onlinelibrary.wiley.com/doi/10.1002/14651858.CD003868.pub2/pdf/standard> (accessed 20 April 2013).

Neurolytic blocking agents

Subhash Jain

Neurolytic agents 32
    Introduction 32
    Types of neurolytic agents 32
    Absolute alcohol 33
    Phenol 34
    Glycerol 36
Selection of a neurolytic agent 37
    Intrathecal (subarachnoid) injection 37
    Phenol and hyperbaricity 37
    Alcohol and hypobaricity 37
    Patient position post injection 38
Conclusion 39
    Key learning points 39
Further reading 40

Neurolytic agents

Introduction

The pain of approximately 90% of cancer patients can be managed using pharmacological agents such as opiates, non-opiates, and adjuvants. In developed and developing countries where opiates are scarce or very expensive, neurolysis may be an appropriate choice. Neurolytic nerve blocks are achieved using a number of chemical agents which produce a long-lasting impact on neural fibres. The block reduces intractable pain caused by tumour invasion of soft tissues, nerves, or various organs.

The use of neurolytic agents, such as alcohol, phenol, glycerol, and ammonium compounds, in various concentrations and at various sites in the body, has proved that the idea of achieving adequate analgesia without attendant side effects is difficult. Enough damage needs to be done to the nerve to produce the changes of Wallerian degeneration. Cautious use of neurolytic agents in carefully selected patients who have given fully informed consent is, therefore, essential.

Types of neurolytic agents

There are several neurolytic agents/techniques currently used for interrupting axonal conduction (Table 3.1). Those commonly used include absolute ethyl alcohol, phenol, ammonium sulphate, silver nitrate, and chlorocresol.

Table 3.1 Showing neurolytic agents/techniques and their pros and cons

Agent	Advantages	Disadvantages
Alcohol (50–100%)	Hypobaricity useful in some cases	Neuritis; solution may spread beyond area desired, can cause sloughing of superficial areas
Phenol (6–12% in saline, glycerine, or contrast dye)	Hyperbaricity of glycerine solutions useful in some cases	Less profound and shorter duration block than alcohol; neuritis, although probably less than alcohol; solution may spread beyond area desired, can cause sloughing of superficial areas
Cryotherapy	Reversible, no neuritis, small area of destruction	Very exact probe placement required, large probe needed (12–14 gauge)
Radiofrequency	Small area of destruction	Neuritis can occur, very accurate probe placement required, large probe needed (16–18 gauge)

Absolute alcohol

Absolute alcohol is available as ethyl alcohol. Alcohol is available in the US as a 1mL single-dose ampoule. In the UK it is available as a 5mL ampoule. It is irritating to local tissues and causes considerable temporary pain during injection. The pre-injection of a local anaesthetic prevents this. Absolute alcohol is volatile, hygroscopic, and absorbs moisture from the atmosphere, so its contents should be used immediately after the ampoule is opened. The burning produced by alcohol is due to a direct effect on muscles and other tissues. The initial action is a local anaesthetic effect; later, there is a destructive action on nerve tissue.

Absolute alcohol is commonly used as a neurolytic agent for peripheral nerve block (see Table 3.2), cranial nerve block (trigeminal nerve), and sympathetic blocks. This drug is hypobaric to cerebrospinal fluid (CSF). Because the solution is lighter than the CSF, the painful side must be uppermost when it is injected into the subarachnoid space. A small volume of alcohol is used for neurolytic blocks and thus produces none of the systemic side effects as of ingested ethanol.

The alcohol produces a non-selective neuronal destruction. It is thought that its neurolytic action is through dehydration of the nerve tissues, extraction of cholesterol, phospholipids, and cerebrosides. Furthermore, it affects myelin sheath, causing precipitation of mucoprotein and lipoprotein. The uptake of alcohol by neural tissue is rapid. When injected into the subarachnoid space, only 10% is present in the CSF after 10 minutes. A typical response to alcohol injection in neural tissue includes myelin sheath disruption and inflammatory responses, followed by demyelination and degeneration. Subarachnoid alcohol injection leads to degeneration of axis cylinders in the posterior root. The posterior root ganglion near the level of injection shows moderate swelling and chromatolysis, followed by intracellular oedema and finally Wallerian degeneration. When alcohol is injected, extreme care is required to avoid any local tissue injury or infiltration to prevent cellulitis or necrosis of adjacent tissues. After the injection, the needle

Table 3.2 Experimental use of ethanol as a neurolytic agent in peripheral nerves

Study (year)	Concentration of alcohol (%)	Result
Finkelberg (1907)	60–80	Persistent paralysis
May (1912)	76, 80, 90, 100	Motor paralysis
	50	No motor paralysis
Gordon (1914)	80	Progressive motor paralysis
Nasaroff (1925)	70	Incomplete and temporary paralysis
Labat (1933)	48 (with 1% procaine), 95	No demonstrable difference in paralysis
Labat and Greene (1931)	33	No paresis or paralysis

should be flushed with a local anaesthetic or normal saline solution to avoid depositing residual alcohol along the needle track.

The most common problems after alcohol injection are post-injection neuritis, hyperaesthesia, paraesthesia, and persistent pain at the site of the injection. When used for coeliac or lumbar sympathetic neurolysis, postural hypotension may occur after the block.

Phenol

In 1867 Lister introduced the use of phenol as an antiseptic. Phenol is also known as carbolic acid and has local anaesthetic properties when it is used in low concentration. Phenol is the most commonly used neurolytic agent in treating intractable pain (see history of use in Table 3.3). Putnam and Hampton used phenol by injection for neurolysis. Maher deserves credit for the application of phenol as a neurolytic agent. Nathan and Scott reported that phenol produced a dual action. The initial blockade produced by phenol is believed to be a conduction blockade similar to a reversible local anaesthetic block. Unlike alcohol, phenol injection therefore is much less painful. However, the neurolytic action on nerve fibres then leads to an irreversible conduction blockade.

Phenol or carbolic acid is a benzene ring with one hydroxyl group substituted for a hydrogen ion. In its pure state, phenol is colourless and poorly soluble, forming a 6.7% solution in water. On exposure to air, phenol oxidizes to form quinones and other derivatives that give it a reddish tinge. Phenol is highly soluble in glycerine. At higher concentrations, phenol causes tissue injury, protein coagulation, and necrosis. It is excreted by the kidneys as various conjugated derivatives.

Phenol causes indiscriminate destruction depending on its concentration. Iggo and Walsh showed a selective block of smaller nerve fibres using phenol 5%. Nathan and colleagues reported that phenol first blocked the non-myelinated C fibres and then thinly myelinated A delta fibres. Pedersen and Juu-Jensen reported that the motor effect of intrathecal phenol solution was a result of indiscriminate fibre damage. The primary neurolytic effect appears to be the result of protein degeneration and non-selective destruction. The maximal degeneration occurs at 2 weeks and maximal destruction at 14 weeks. The effect of 5% phenol is equivalent to that of 40% alcohol.

Although phenol is not available commercially in an injectable form, it can be prepared by the hospital pharmacy. The solution can be in water in the concentration range from 4–6%. The phenol is prepared in glycerine as a hyperbaric solution ranging from 4–10%. It is released from glycerine slowly; this is advantageous when used as an intrathecal agent. Because of its hyperbaric nature, spread can be controlled, and thus it will have a localized effect. For selected cases of spasticity, a higher concentration of phenol 20% in glycerine can be used. When injected in non-neural tissues, the aqueous phenol solution is a strong sclerotic agent. This drug also may be dissolved in radio-contrast dye, providing a hyperbaric radiopaque solution. The various properties of alcohol and phenol are shown in Table 3.4.

Table 3.3 History of use of phenol as neurolytic agent

Study (year)	Application
Nechaev (1933)	Local anaesthesia
Putnam and Hampton (1936)	Gasserian ganglion neurolysis
Mandl (1947)	Chemical sympathectomy
Haxton (1949)	Paravertebral injection for intermittent claudication
Maher (1955)	Intrathecal injection for cancer pain
Kelly and Gautier-Smith (1959)	Intrathecal injection for spasticity of upper motor neuron disease
Nathan (1959)	Intrathecal injection for spasticity of paraplegia
Nathan and Sears (1960)	Effects on nerve conduction in cat spinal nerve roots
Iggo and Walsh (1960)	Blockade of fibres in cat spinal nerve roots

Table 3.4 Comparison of alcohol and phenol

Property	Phenol	Alcohol
Physical properties	Clear, colourless, pungent odour Poorly soluble in water Unstable at room temperature Hyperbaric relative to cerebrospinal fluid	Clear, colourless Absorbs water on exposure to air Stable at room temperature Hypobaric relative to cerebrospinal fluid
Chemical structure	Acid	Alcohol
Concentrations (%)	6–10	50–100
Equipotent neurolytic concentration (%)	5	40
Complications of use in neurolysis	Neuritis (uncommon) Toxicity at higher doses Hepatic and cardiac complications	Neuritis (common) Toxicity at commonly used doses
Sites of use (listed in order of preference)	Epidural Paravertebral Peripheral nerve roots Intrathecal Cranial nerves	Intrathecal Coeliac ganglion Lumbar sympathetic chain Cranial nerves Paravertebral Epidural (low concentrations)

Glycerol

Earlier reports on the use of glycerol for relieving pain of trigeminal neuralgia generated widespread interest in its use. Histopathological examination revealed extensive myelin sheath swelling, axonolysis, and severe inflammatory response after intraneuronal injection. Electron microscopy confirmed Wallerian degeneration, phagocytosis, and mast cell degranulation. The differential effects of various concentrations of glycerol have been studied in experimental models, but no histological data are available to support these observations.

Selection of a neurolytic agent

Physical characteristics of the two more commonly used neurolytic agents make them suitable for two different subgroups of patients (see Table 3.4). Alcohol, on the one hand, is hypobaric and can be injected with the patient prone. Thus, it is suitable for a patient who is unable to lie supine owing to pain. Hyperbaric phenol, on the other hand, can reach dorsal nerve roots of a supine patient after intrathecal injection. Jacob and Howland found a higher incidence of sphincter impairment with alcohol injection than with phenol. In cases of intractable pain, however, analgesic efficacy was equal for the agents. Phenol in glycerine is hyperbaric and diffuses out very slowly. Therefore, its neurolytic action can be controlled by adjusting patient position at the time of injection. Alcohol has a quicker onset of action, but its site of action can be controlled in the vertical neuraxis by tilting the table head to foot or to one side.

Intrathecal (subarachnoid) injection

The technique of subarachnoid administration of neurolytic agents was used first by Maher, who advocated the use of phenol as an intrathecal neurolytic drug. Various authors reported good relief of pain in 65–70% of cases after a subarachnoid injection of phenol. Maher recommended the use of phenol in glycerine as the drug of choice because it is hyperbaric, minimally diffusible, provides a slow release of phenol, and has a low incidence of complications. Brown reported unsatisfactory results with subarachnoid phenol in patients with chronic pain of benign origin, and Mark and his associates confirmed that malignant pain responds better than chronic benign pain. Papo and Visca reported a high failure rate and poor results with cervical and thoracic subarachnoid neurolytic blocks. The duration of relief induced by subarachnoid phenol varies from <1 month to 10 months. Mehta reported a higher success rate when the pain was present for <4 months before the block was administered. Overall, properly selected patients and techniques are mandatory to provide good quality pain relief in a high proportion of patients.

Phenol and hyperbaricity

Phenol in glycerine is advantageous when the painful site can be placed in a dependent position to take advantage of the hyperbaric nature of the solution. The diffusion of this solution is slow and the local site of action can be controlled easily. Maher found that 1mL of phenol in glycerine can treat three nerve roots adequately. The slow release of phenol allows its destructive action to be well controlled in the desired dermatomal distribution.

Alcohol and hypobaricity

Alcohol is a hypobaric solution without the localized effect of phenol. Injected into the subarachnoid space, the solution can disperse caudal or cephalad. When alcohol is used, the painful side must be kept upward. This drug has other disadvantages as a neurolytic drug for subarachnoid use. The analgesic effect is not attained for several days, and the chance of tissue sloughing is greater with alcohol than with phenol. Alcohol neuritis is a well-known phenomenon that may occur when alcohol is injected near a somatic nerve. The burning pain caused by alcohol may be worse than the original pain.

Patient position post injection

Whichever neurolytic agent is used, the position of the patient should be retained for approximately 45 minutes after injection to allow the neurolytic agent to become fixed to the nerve roots.

Conclusion

Key learning points
- Where access to conventional medical management is limited, one-off neurolytic blocks may provide months of pain relief.
- It is vital to fully inform patients regarding numbness, weakness, dysaesthetic pain, or sensations which can arise as a result of neurolytic blocks.
- Following intrathecal neurolysis the position of the patient should be retained for 45 minutes to allow the agent to become fixed to the nervous tissue.

Further reading

Derrick WS (1970). Control of pain in the cancer patient by subarachnoid alcohol block. *Postgrad Med*, **48**, 232–37.

Iggo A, Walsh EG. (1960) Selective block of small fibers in the spinal roots by phenol. *Brain*, **83**, 701–8.

Jacob RG, Howland WS (1966). A comparison of intrathecal alcohol and phenol. *J Ky Med Assoc*, **64**, 40.

Kelly RE, Gautier-Smith PC (1959). Intrathecal phenol in the treatment of reflex spasms and spasticity. *Lancet*, **2**(7112), 1102–5.

Maher RM (1955). Relief of pain in incurable cancer. *Lancet*, **1**, 18–20.

Maher RM (1957). Neurone selection in relief of pain. Further experiences with intrathecal injections. *Lancet*, **1**, 16–19.

Mandl F (1949) *Paravertebral Block*. New York: Grune & Stratton.

Mark VH, White JC, Zervas NT, Ervin FR, Richardson EP (1962). Intrathecal use of phenol for the relief of chronic severe pain. *N Engl J Med*, **262**, 589–93.

Nathan PW (1959) Intrathecal phenol to relieve spasticity in paraplegia. *Lancet*, **2**, 1099–102.

Nathan PW, Sears TA, Smith MC. (1965). Effects of phenol solution on the nerve roots of the cat. An electrophysiological and histological study. *J Neurol Sci*, **2**, 7–29.

Putnam TJ, Hampton AO. (1936). A technique of injection in the gasserian ganglion under roentgenographic control. *Arch Neurol Psychiatry*, **35**, 92–8.

Wood KA (1978). The use of phenol as a neurolytic agent: A review. *Pain*, **5**, 205–29.

The role of surgery in cancer pain management

Paul Eldridge

Types of pain 42
   Introduction 42
   Causes 42
   Palliation 42
Surgical principles in the treatment of cancer pain 44
   Treat the cause 44
   Electrical neuromodulation 45
   Chemical neuromodulation 45
   Neuroablation (lesions) 45
Outcomes 47
   Structural outcome/change 47
   Symptomatic outcome 47
Intractability 48
   WHO analgesic ladder and pitfalls 48
   WHO analgesic ladder or interventional/surgical
      techniques? 48
   Empowering patient choice 49
Conclusion 50
   Key learning points 50
Further reading 51

Types of pain

Introduction

Patients suffering from cancer frequently experience pain, and this may well be the primary presenting symptom. However, it is important to realize that pain associated with cancer may have a number of different aetiologies, and this is often overlooked when analysing the particular situation of a patient, who, in the context of cancer, complains of pain. It is also the case, though not the subject of this chapter, that the psychological state of the patient with a terminal condition is also important.

Cancer pain may be of many types, i.e. related to cancer, its treatment, or pre-existing. It is vital to know the predominant pain and nature of it so as to manage it effectively.

Causes

- Neuropathic—pain deriving from a disorder of the pain pathways within the central or peripheral nervous systems
- Non-metastatic manifestations of systemic cancer
- 'Iatrogenic' post chemotherapy
- 'Iatrogenic' post radiotherapy, e.g. brachial plexopathy
- Nociceptive, e.g. pathological fractures
- Direct invasion of surrounding tissues
- Deformity
- Co-incidental, i.e. pre-existing conditions such as osteoarthritis.

The incidence of the 'iatrogenic' problems noted here are substantially less with modern regimens than historically. It remains, however, of critical importance that the differential diagnosis is correctly made between these possibilities, remembering that they are not exclusive. In the palliative care setting, the emphasis can easily become prioritized towards pain relief 'palliation', and then the treatment needs and possibilities for the original tumour get overlooked; this is increasingly true when multidisciplinary care is involved as it may be difficult to get together all the parties with the relevant imaging and clinical information. This is driven by ever increasing sub-specialization within medicine, and whilst this trend has good justification this issue needs to be accommodated.

Palliation

It is worthwhile to consider the meaning of the term palliation. It does not have, at least in general use, a precise meaning. It can be taken to mean treatment undertaken without the intention of providing a cure of the condition, or a treatment aimed at alleviating symptoms only. However, there are many treatments that whilst not eradicating the disease do 'palliate' by extending life expectancy, and not all treatments aimed at eradicating cancer achieve this.

It is the case now that the prevalence of cancer is increasing because even if the disease cannot be eradicated, considerable increases in life expectancy are achieved; this may well influence the choices made in pain control. It is also the case that specialists in other fields than that of the cancer being treated may not appreciate the nature or scale of these advances.

This is a particular risk in palliative care, or other agency managing pain, especially as these specialities do not themselves manage cancerous conditions. Neurosurgeons are perhaps fortunate in being involved directly in the management of patients with tumours of the nervous system.

The 'accurate' knowledge of prognosis does affect, as you might expect, the choice of treatment option for pain relief.

Surgical principles in the treatment of cancer pain

The surgical principles of treating pain as mentioned in other chapters apply in cancer pain as much as they do in any other situation and these are in the following order:
- Treat the cause
- Electrical neuromodulation
- Chemical neuromodulation
- Neuroablation (lesion).

Treat the cause

The most basic and obvious strategy. Surgery has been the cornerstone of cancer treatments now for many years. There are three objectives to surgery. First to establish a pathological diagnosis, second to attempt to eradicate the tumour, and third to palliate symptoms. Pain is of course only one symptom; broadly speaking the others are encompassed by the concept of loss of function. Surgery may be wholly or partially successful in achieving these objectives; and even in some instances not even a clear diagnosis is achieved.

The diagnosis is important as the pathological type and histological grading in association with the staging of the tumour will most accurately predict the prognosis. This will be important when considering whether resective (sometimes referred to as cytoreductive), lesional, or neuromodulatory techniques are to be considered. Resective surgery will often be accompanied by reconstructive surgery. This may vary from a minimum to quite complex procedures such as spinal fixation after decompressive surgery.

The accuracy of the prognosis is usually adequate to direct treatment choice, but it still remains to a degree an uncertain area.

Specific neurosurgical examples of treating the cause are detailed elsewhere, but perhaps the best example is that of decompressive surgery and fixation for spinal metastatic disease—nicely shown in a randomized prospective trial to improve not only longevity and function but also to provide excellent pain relief. The macroscopic resections performed for primary malignant cerebral tumours—the gliomas—are another example of this strategy.

There have been considerable improvements in surgical technologies, allied with improvements in operative, and perioperative anaesthetic care, together with advances in critical care that have all summated to reduce perioperative morbidity which has made the risk balance of surgery much more favourable. The progress made in surgical techniques towards less and less invasive techniques which can still achieve the same therapeutic objective is clear to all; in addition tumour treatments using chemotherapeutic agents, and specialized radiation techniques have also advanced.

Consequently survival times for cancerous conditions have improved, so has the general health of the population so that more elderly patients can now be considered for more extensive surgical procedures. In other words, the prevalence of cancer has increased substantially.

Electrical neuromodulation

For surgical purposes there are two means to neuromodulate the nervous system. One is by electrical stimulation, and the other by drug delivery systems. In both cases the goal is to deliver the treatment to a specific target thereby avoiding unwanted side effects.

The specific target chosen for treatment of pain is clearly critical and will of course involve the pain pathways. In general the same targets will be under consideration for lesional techniques and it is easy to see how an electrode providing stimulation can be substituted for a lesion. The advantage should be reversibility, better longevity of treatment, less loss of function, and the absence of secondary dysaesthetic pain syndromes. However, electrical stimulation has more often been used for neuropathic pain rather than nociceptive pain. The most widely used technique of spinal cord stimulation is not felt to be effective for nociceptive pain, the type of pain common in the pain of cancer. Nevertheless, there may be a case in the future for revisiting this area, particularly in consideration of deep brain targets.

Chemical neuromodulation

The nervous system functions at a synaptic level chemically rather than electrically; hence the targeting of drugs taken systemically is by designing or choosing the molecule to be active only at certain receptors. The nervous system itself achieves specificity of action by only activating relevant synapses so that only at this physical point is the relevant chemical transmitter abundant. Thus the goal of drug delivery systems is to improve on systemic administration, which must of necessity include the whole body. For practical purposes this means intrathecal drug delivery systems, and the improvement in specificity for most drugs is approximation at best. Thus the 'effective' dose of morphine equivalent to an intrathecal dose will be approximately 100× more than that given systemically for the same analgesic effect. Although this is nowhere near the specificity achieved by the nervous system itself it is a vast improvement on systemic administration. In addition to avoiding side effects this level of dosage can improve the efficacy of a drug by providing a higher concentration of drug at its point of action than could ever be achieved by oral or parenteral administration; partly this is due to issues of absorption, and partly as it enables the drug to be delivered beyond certain physiological barriers, such as the blood–brain barrier.

Neuroablation (lesions)

Although current neurosurgical practice is to avoid lesioning wherever possible this course of action finds a relative exception in cancer pain. This reluctance to lesion the nervous system for pain arises because the longevity of lesional techniques is limited—often to around 12–18 months—and because they carry a feared side effect of inducing a new dysaesthetic pain caused by the lesion itself, and these syndromes are typically refractory to treatment. However, in a palliative context these considerations are less relevant because the progression of the patient's disease means there is insufficient time for these complications to occur. However this issue—the longevity of lesional techniques—may need to be revisited as survival times with cancers improve. The data regarding the longevity and incidence of dysaesthetic problems of many lesional techniques is historical, and comes only from case series. This is because of the relatively rapid demise of patients with cancer, and hence few outcomes beyond even 6 months.

Outcomes

This is an area of considerable importance; it can be considered in two ways. The structural changes brought about by an intervention and the resulting effect on the patient's symptomatology and quality of life.

Structural outcome/change

The structural outcome of the intervention should be possible to measure with higher-quality preoperative and postoperative investigations: most obviously imaging but perhaps also neurophysiological assessment of the size and nature of a lesion that has actually been created prior to re-evaluating this area. This concept can be extended to the other classes of treatment including 'treat the cause' and neuromodulation—in the second example neurophysiological techniques may be more prominent. There is an argument for making post-procedural verification of a treatment intervention mandatory to establish good quality control.

Symptomatic outcome

It is critically important to be able to measure the symptomatic outcomes of treatment (which should include outcomes of those in whom interventions are *not* undertaken). This is both difficult and demanding. It is difficult as it can be a challenge to measure in a quantitative manner quality of life, not just simply pain relief; demanding because the data can be time-consuming to collect in a complete manner. However, it would seem wrong to carry out major invasive procedures without being able to understand outcomes. A commissioner of healthcare could and should demand that a potential provider be able to give this information as a condition of using that provider of service.

Intractability

WHO analgesic ladder and pitfalls

The WHO treatment ladder has been in practice for many years. Within it is the concept of intractability, before treatment is 'escalated' to the level of interventions. There is now an argument to update the ladder and to reconsider the logic behind it.

The concept of intractability is almost universally employed in consideration of medical therapies, and in the context that an invasive surgical procedure should not be contemplated under any circumstances until intractability has been demonstrated. However, 'intractability' is not quantitatively defined. It depends not only on the efficacy of the treatment but also on the impact of side effects from the medication. There are a variety of qualitative measures mainly to do with quality of life such as the EuroQuol 5D which attempt to measure this, and from their qualitative scales a quantitative variable is derived employed most notably by the National Institute for Health and Care Excellence (NICE) in trying to relate costs of treatment or intervention to benefit derived in terms of quality of life, and from this economic information make decisions regarding funding of interventions. Nevertheless, all admit the shortcomings of this approach and its relative insensitivity to reductions in quality of life in certain situations.

A particular issue is the understanding of the side effects of medications, particularly but not only those affecting cognition. Two good examples of this are the comparison, in a randomized trial, of best medical management against intrathecal drug treatment of pain which found that quality of life and survival were improved in the interventional group as much as a result of the side effects of the medical treatments, and a similar result in a trial of surgical intervention for metastatic spinal disease.

The WHO ladder follows the traditional medical model in which it is presumed that non-invasive medical (pharmacological) treatments should be exhausted at all costs before a surgical treatment is embarked upon. This is based on the perception that surgical morbidity, side effects, and complications are far more frequent and significant than is in fact the case.

WHO analgesic ladder or interventional/surgical techniques?

- An alternative way to prioritize interventional or surgical techniques is to consider that they are ideal for dealing with focal pathologies; and that when successful and after recovery are free from side effects, unlike medical treatments where side effects are dose-related and therefore perpetual.
- Surgical and anaesthetic techniques have now substantially advanced, leading to less invasive treatments and shorter hospital stays as perioperative care improves; this of course improves the balance between risk and benefit in favour of benefit.
- This is well illustrated by the two randomized trials referenced earlier, and these should be regarded as Class 1 evidence.

Empowering patient choice

- There is accordingly a good case for revising the WHO treatment ladder with this in mind, and also to empower the patient in this area of decision-making.
- The argument here is that at the point of diagnosis the patient should be made aware of the natural history of a condition, all the potential treatments available including interventions, and the final duty of the physician is to make a recommendation.
- It is the case that in addition to case volume, the ability of a centre to provide all possible treatments results in improved outcomes.

Conclusion

There are a number of procedures available within the neurosurgical armamentarium for the control of cancer pain, including surgical treatment of
cancer. Whilst in the main cancer pain is successfully controlled by medical
means, the neurosurgical methods, and in particular the lesional techniques,
should not be abandoned and probably have a greater place than has been
appreciated; the ability to achieve significant pain relief, without large doses
of opioids, may well result in improved quality of life and, by itself, improved
survival.

Key learning points

- Treating the cancer by itself can be very effective in controlling pain.
- Close collaboration between disease-specific specialty, medical and
  radiation oncology, palliative care, functional neurosurgery, and pain
  medicine is vital to achieve good outcomes.
- At the point of diagnosis, the patient has a right to be given full
  information concerning prognosis, and to be fully informed concerning
  all potential treatment options, interventional as well as medical, in
  order to be able to make a fully informed choice, and to decide for
  themselves the point of intractability.

Further reading

Bittar RG, Kar-Purkayastha I, Owen SL, Bear RE, Green A, Wang S, et al. (2005). Deep brain stimulation for pain relief: a meta-analysis. *Journal of Clinical Neuroscience*, **12**(5), 515–19.

Cetas JS, Raslan A, Burchiel KJ (2011). Evidence base for destructive procedures. In Winn HR (ed) *Youmans Neurological Surgery*, 6th edn, pp. 1835–44. Philadelphia, PA: Elsevier.

Freeman WJ, Watts JW (1948). Psychosurgery for pain. *South Med J*, **41**, 1045–9.

Jones B, Finlay I, Ray A, Simpson B (2003). Is there still a role for open cordotomy in cancer pain management? *J Pain Symptom Manag*, **25**, 179–84.

Leksell L (1951). The stereotaxic method and radiosurgery of the brain *Acta Chir Scand*, **102**, 312–9.

Lihua P, Su M, Zejun Z, Ke W, Bennett MI (2013). Spinal cord stimulation for cancer-related pain in adults. *Cochrane Database Syst Rev*, **2**, CD009389. doi: 10.1002/14651858.CD009389.pub2.

Morrica G (1974). Chemical hypophysectomy for cancer pain. In Bonica JJ (ed) *Advances in Neurology*, Vol. 4, pp. 707–14. New York: Raven Press.

Nauta HJ, Soukup VM, Fabian RH, Lin JT, Grady JJ, Williams CG, et al. (2000). Punctate midline myelotomy for the relief of visceral cancer pain. *J Neurosurg*, **92**(2), 125–30.

Patchell RA, Tibbs PA, Regine WF, Payne R, Saris S, Kryscio RJ, et al. (2005). Direct decompressive surgical resection in the treatment of spinal cord compression caused by metastatic cancer: a randomised trial. *Lancet*, **366**(9486), 643–8.

Raslan AM, Cetas JS, McCartney S, Burchiel KJ (2011). Destructive procedures for control of cancer pain: the case for cordotomy. *J Neurosurg*, **114**(1), 155–70.

Schug SA, Zech D, Dörr U (1990). Cancer pain management according to WHO analgesic guidelines. *J Pain Symptom Manag*, **5**, 27–32.

Smith TJ, Staats PS, Deer T, Stearns LJ, Rauck RL, Boortz-Marx RL, et al.; Implantable Drug Delivery Systems Study Group (2002). Randomized clinical trial of an implantable drug delivery system compared with comprehensive medical management for refractory cancer pain: impact on pain, drug-related toxicity, and survival. *J Clin Oncol*, **20**(19), 4040–9.

Thomas KC, Nosyk B, Fisher CG, Dvorak M, Patchell RA, Regine WF, et al. (2006). Cost-effectiveness of surgery plus radiotherapy versus radiotherapy alone for metastatic epidural spinal cord compression. *Int J Radiat Oncol Biol Phys*, **66**(4), 1212–18.

Yen CP, Kung SS, Su YF, Lin WC, Howng SL, Kwan AL (2005). Stereotactic bilateral anterior cingulotomy for intractable pain. *J Clin Neurosci*, **12**(8), 886–90.

Oncological management of cancer pain

Chinnamani Eswar

Introduction 54
    Systemic treatments 54
    Chemotherapy 54
    Hormones 54
    Targeted agents 54
    Bisphosphonates 55
Locoregional treatments 56
    Radiotherapy 56
    Radioisotopes 57
    Surgery 57
Conclusion 58
    Key learning points 58
Further reading 59

Introduction

Systemic treatments

Appropriate and timely oncological management of the primary tumour and secondaries can result in a significant improvement of pain. The treatment given is often palliative aimed at rapid symptom relief and needs to be combined with pharmacological and non-pharmacological measures of pain control. Cancer treatment can either be systemic in the form of chemotherapy, hormones, and targeted agents or locoregional in the form of radiotherapy and surgery.

Chemotherapy

- Chemotherapy is given intravenously or orally and travels systemically, working both on the primary tumour and distant metastases.
- When patients respond to treatment there is a decrease in volume of the tumour, often resulting in pain relief.
- In some tumour types such as small cell cancers there can be a rapid symptomatic response within days but in most other tumour types it could take 4–6 weeks before observing any symptomatic response.
- The decision to use chemotherapy as a palliative treatment is made after a careful assessment of the patient, balancing the treatment benefits against the treatment-related toxicity.
- Haematological malignancies such as lymphoma and myeloma are other examples where chemotherapy can result in pain relief due to rapid effect on the malignant cells.

Hormones

Hormonal agents play an important role in the management of many cancers. Metastatic prostate cancer with widespread bone metastases is a good example where antiandrogens and luteinizing hormone-releasing hormone (LHRH) agonists induce a rapid anticancer response with good pain relief occurring within days. The response from first-line hormonal treatment also continues, often, lasting 2–3 years. Similarly in oestrogen receptor-positive breast cancer with bone metastases several lines of hormonal agents (tamoxifen, aromatase inhibitors, exemestane) can be used in sequence over many years providing good pain relief.

Targeted agents

Over the last 5 years several new targeted agents have come into clinical use. For example, in metastatic renal cell cancer new targeted agents such as the multikinase inhibitors (sunitinib, sorafenib) have been shown in large randomized studies to have a good response on the primary and areas of bone metastasis thereby helping in achieving good pain control. There are several other agents currently in use in lung cancer, melanoma, breast cancer, bowel cancer, and other tumour types.

Bisphosphonates

When given alongside other local and systemic therapies bisphosphonates have proven benefit in decreasing pain from bone metastasis. They also decrease the number of skeletal events such as pathological fractures and spinal cord compression due to vertebral collapse and thereby help in improved pain control. The newer generation of drugs such as zoledronate and denosumab are very effective and have very few side effects.

Locoregional treatments

Radiotherapy

- External beam radiotherapy is delivered by linear accelerators which produce mega voltage x-rays. They are very precisely focused on the primary or secondary tumour with adequate margins using modern radiotherapy planning and treatment equipment. This precision in treatment delivery helps to achieve a good tumour response and rapid pain relief while reducing toxicity by avoiding involvement of adjacent normal structures in the treatment field.
- For areas of bone metastasis causing pain, several studies have confirmed that a single treatment of 8Gy planned and treated on the same day provides a simple and effective way of reducing pain.
- Around 80% of patients achieve effective pain relief with palliative radiotherapy and the pain relief can start within a week but the maximum benefit is seen in about 4 weeks.
- However, it can take up to 12 weeks for complete healing of the involved bone. Although radiotherapy is usually not repeated in the same area an 8Gy single fraction can be repeated if there is a relapse of pain after a durable period of response.
- Pathological fractures and areas of vertebral collapse causing spinal cord compression or nerve root compression can be again treated by a single fraction or a course of radiotherapy. This helps to reduce tumour volume and stabilize the affected bone and thereby helps to reduce the pain.
- Radiotherapy is also very effective in controlling pain due to primary or secondary tumours locally invading into adjacent structures. A course of radiotherapy in these cases helps to shrink the tumour mass and relieves the pressure on invading structures.
- Some common scenarios are primary lung tumours invading into chest wall, vertebrae, or mediastinum.
- Severe headache from a brain metastases invading into brain tissue and causing raised intracranial pressure can be relieved by a course of palliative radiotherapy.
- Locally advanced breast cancer invading through the chest wall and brachial plexus can be treated by a course of treatment for pain relief.
- In patients with widespread bone metastases, mainly in prostate and breast cancer, sometimes large areas are treated with a single fraction or a course of radiotherapy.
- Common examples are treating the whole of the pelvis or hemi pelvis in a single field which can help with immediate pain relief and help to improve the quality of life. But during these treatments patients are often commenced on steroids and antiemetics to prevent treatment-induced nausea and flu-like symptoms.

Radioisotopes

- In patients with widespread bone metastases with generalized pain, localized external beam radiotherapy or even large field treatment will not be able to encompass regions of pain.
- One approach in this situation would be to use radionuclides given intravenously which are bone seeking. They are physiologically attracted to areas of bone mineralization where they work and help in controlling the pain.
- Strontium was the main isotope used until recently but a new agent Xofigo® (formerly called Alpharadin®) with a shorter half-life has been shown to have significant benefit in metastatic castrate-resistant prostate cancer in a multicentre randomized trial. Baseline blood counts are routinely checked prior to administration due to risk of bone marrow suppression.

Surgery

- Although major surgery is usually not indicated in patients with metastatic cancer some palliative surgical procedures can provide rapid pain relief.
- In pathological fractures internal fixation can help with pain control and can help to restore mobility.
- Urgent spinal stabilization in patients with vertebral collapse is another example where restoration of the skeletal structure helps.
- In patients with primary or secondary brain tumours local invasion can result in obstructive hydrocephalus, causing severe headache which needs surgical decompression.
- Toilet mastectomy, ascitic drainage, and oesophageal stent insertion are all examples of how surgical procedures can help with pain relief.
- Palliative radiotherapy is often combined with these surgical procedures to achieve better results.

Conclusion

Cancer-related pain usually needs a multimodal approach in its management. In addition to the immediate use of analgesic support the patient needs a careful assessment by the oncologist with a multidisciplinary team discussion exploring all possible oncological treatments. There also needs to be involvement of the patient with clear discussion on the pros and cons of each approach. The focus in all this has to be immediate symptom relief without worsening the patient's quality of life.

Key learning points

- Understanding the importance of the role of systemic treatments such as chemotherapy, hormones, and targeted agents in cancer pain relief.
- Understanding the importance of the role of palliative radiotherapy and radioisotopes in cancer pain management.
- Understanding the importance of the role of surgery and supportive treatments such as bisphosphonates in pain relief.
- Understanding the importance of a multidisciplinary approach in cancer pain management.

Further reading

Dennis K, Makhani L, Zeng L, Lam H, Chow E (2013). Single fraction conventional external beam radiation therapy for bone metastases: a systematic review of randomised controlled trials. *Radiother Oncol*, **106**(1), 5–14.

Janjan N (2001). Bone metastases: approaches to management. *Semin Oncol*, **28**(11), 28–34.

Ripamonti CI, Bandieri E, Roila F (2011). Management of cancer pain: ESMO Clinical Practice Guidelines, On behalf of the ESMO Guidelines Working Group. *Ann Oncol*, **22**(6), vi69–vi77.

Rosen LS, Gordon D, Kaminski M, Howell A, Belch A, Mackey J, *et al.* (2001). Zoledronic acid versus pamidronate in the treatment of skeletal metastases in patients with breast cancer or osteolytic lesions of multiple myeloma: a phase III, double blind, comparative trial. *Cancer J*, **7**(5), 377–87.

Salazar OM, Sandhu T, da Motta NW, Escutia MA, Lanzós-Gonzales E, Mouelle-Sone A, *et al.* (2001). Fractionated half-body irradiation (HBI) for the rapid palliation of widespread, symptomatic, metastatic bone disease: a randomized Phase III trial of the International Atomic Energy Agency (IAEA). *Int J Radiat Oncol Biol Phys*, **50**(3), 765–75.

Chapter 6

Pelvic pain

Arun Bhaskar

Introduction 62
Case discussion 63
   History 63
   Disease progression 63
   Initial care in community 63
   Initial care in specialist pain clinic 64
   Disease progression and palliative care management 64
   Further management in specialist pain clinic 64
   Further disease progression (sacral pain) 65
   End of life care in palliative care setting 65
Conclusion 67
   Key learning points 67
Further reading 68

Introduction

Pelvic pain in patients with malignancy can be debilitating and has a significant impact on survival and subsequent quality of life. A meta-analysis showed a pooled pain prevalence of 52% with urogenital malignancy, 60% with gynaecological malignancy, and 59% in those with gastrointestinal malignancy. Pain can be due to the tumour invading the deep tissues by stretching or distending hollow viscus as well as compressing it; the tissues could also be damaged due to surgery or radiotherapy. Patients would be experiencing autonomic disturbances like urinary retention and/or faecal incontinence; some patients would already have had a diversion procedure like urostomy and colostomy as part of their pelvic clearance surgery. The mobility could also be affected due to tumour involvement of the lumbosacral plexus as well as oedema of the lower limbs due to occlusion of lymphatic and venous drainage. Many patients find it difficult to cope and require psychological support along with good analgesia during end of life care.

Case discussion

History

- A 34-year-old lady was diagnosed with squamous cell carcinoma of the cervix 2 years after the birth of her first child.
- She underwent total abdominal hysterectomy and bilateral salpingo-oophorectomy along with pelvic and omental lymph node sampling.
- The patient underwent adjuvant chemotherapy, followed by pelvic brachytherapy using vault caesium.
- The patient was on regular follow-up and her condition remained stable.
- She had occasional pain deep in her pelvis, which responded to paracetamol, ibuprofen, and tramadol as required.

Disease progression

- The patient developed symptoms of tenesmus and occasional bleeding per rectum 18 months later and a follow-up scan showed a right-sided pelvic recurrence as a rectosigmoid mass.
- The patient had been complaining of decreased appetite as well as weight loss during this time.
- She underwent surgery, but the tumour was unresectable and she underwent debulking of the tumour as well as a colostomy.
- This was followed-up with further chemotherapy as well as 15 fractions of external beam radiotherapy to the pelvis.
- However, the patient started developing pain in her right leg thought to be due to tumour infiltration of her right lumbosacral plexus.
- The patient also had been complaining of continuing pelvic pain including tenesmus pain and pain in her bladder area associated with micturition.

Initial care in community

- The community palliative care team was involved in her care and she was initially started on slow release morphine 10mg twice daily (12-hourly MR morphine sulphate) as her regular analgesia and morphine sulfate solution 5–10mg (IR morphine) for breakthrough pain, which she was taking about six to eight times a day, but still had been struggling with uncontrolled pain.
- She had both spontaneous and breakthrough pain as well as incident pain (whilst mobilizing and also whilst passing urine).
- The background opioid medication dose was subsequently increased including the dose of the breakthrough pain medications. The slow release morphine dose had now increased to 240mg twice a day with morphine sulfate solution dose to 80mg for rescue analgesia; this analgesic regimen was causing her drowsiness and she was still complaining of severe pain.
- She was started on oral ketamine 10mg four times a day, but this was also not well tolerated as it made her quite delirious and confused.
- She was subsequently switched to a syringe driver delivering subcutaneous diamorphine at a dose of 360mg over 24 hours and was referred to the pain service to look into interventional pain control options.

Initial care in specialist pain clinic

- The patient was started on neuropathic analgesics, i.e. pregabalin and amitriptyline, but these were discontinued because of side effects.
- The patient was started on escitalopram for being low in mood.
- The patient was encouraged to have regular paracetamol at a dose of 1g four times a day.
- We added buccal fentanyl as first-line analgesia for breakthrough pain starting at 100 micrograms and was subsequently titrated to 200 micrograms per episode; she was advised to use 20mg oxycodone as second line and was taken off the diamorphine infusion and reverted back to her long-acting oxycodone dose 80mg twice daily.
- In addition, the patient underwent a caudal epidural block and ganglion impar block (trans-sacrococcygeal approach).
- She had good analgesia following this with significant reduction in her sacral and buttock pain as well as the tenesmus pain.
- The patient did not require additional rescue analgesia for 72 hours, but then started complaining of the return of the tenesmus pain; we carried out radiofrequency ablation (RFA) of the ganglion impar and this helped over the next 3 months.

Disease progression and palliative care management

- The patient did not have any major pain issues for another 3 months and she was started on palliative chemotherapy during this time.
- She noticed difficulty in initiating micturition as well as getting spasmodic pains whilst passing urine.
- The oncologist started her on antispasmodics (Buscopan®) and antibiotics (trimethoprim) as she had developed urinary infection possibly related to retention.
- She was catheterized for this, but an ultrasound scan revealed left-sided hydronephrosis due to tumour infiltration of the left ureter; this was relieved by inserting an ureteric stent and though the constant ache she was feeling in her loin settled a bit, she was still complaining of painful bladder spasms as well as occasional episodes of sharp shooting pain down her left buttock particularly whilst sitting down.

The patient was feeling quite depressed by the fact that she was starting to lose control of her bowel and bladder functions, but also that there had been tumour progression as evidenced by follow-up CT scan despite being on palliative chemotherapy. The patient also found that taking rescue analgesia in the form of oxycodone was making her drowsy and dizzy. Further up-titration of buccal fentanyl to 400 micrograms was not very effective.

Further management in specialist pain clinic

- It was decided that the patient might benefit from a superior hypogastric plexus blockade as the spasmodic pelvic pain seemed to be sympathetically mediated in nature.
- The patient was still undergoing chemotherapy and was not keen to disrupt it; so it was decided to proceed directly to a neurolytic procedure at the same sitting as the diagnostic block to maximize the window of opportunity between cycles of chemotherapy.

- There was the left-sided pelvic mass, hence, it was decided to proceed via a right L5/S1 trans-discal approach.

Following the procedure, the patient did not have any complications and had good analgesia. Additionally the opioid analgesic requirements reduced considerably.

Further disease progression (sacral pain)

Despite having palliative chemotherapy the patient had rapid disease progression with metastasis in the liver as well as sacral involvement of the tumour; this caused severe pain on the left buttock. The patient had further increase in the size of the pelvic mass and this was infiltrating the sacral nerves on both sides.

The interventional options were percutaneous cordotomy, indwelling intrathecal line with an implanted system, and more localized interventions like neurolytic saddle-block with hyperbaric phenol in glycerol. The patient was not very keen on percutaneous cordotomy and we also felt that it may not be the best option as she now had pain in both her buttocks. The option of implanted intrathecal drug delivery system was also deemed inappropriate due to the presence of her stoma and rapid loss of weight including frequent urinary retention and infections.

We carried out bilateral sacral sensory pulsed radiofrequency (RF) and were added using 0.3mL of 6% aqueous phenol through each RF needle port after the RF lesioning. This was preferred over the saddle-block with hyperbaric phenol as it gave a better option to cover the radicular pain on the S1–S2 territory without comprising her ability to mobilize with minimal support. The patient had adequate analgesia, so much so that she could sit down without too much discomfort. She was able to lie down for ten fractions of external beam radiotherapy to her sacrum and pelvis. This was predominantly meant for controlling her bone pain as a palliative measure.

End of life care in palliative care setting

By this time, the patient was getting increasingly low in her mood as she was disappointed that the tumour growth and spread were not being controlled by any of the treatment options. Some of these psychological distresses were perceived as pain by the community team and the patient was once again started on a diamorphine/midazolam syringe driver. This brought up the expected side effects of drowsiness and increased somnolence which resulted in poor intake of oral feeds and fluids. The patient was in a state where she felt tired most of the day, but had periods when she was lucid and expressed her desire to spend her time on a holiday with her 5-year-old daughter and her husband.

We discussed with the patient and her family the option of an indwelling intrathecal line to deliver analgesia and it was decided that we should use an external pump (dedicated intrathecal syringe-driver) due to patient preference and also the advanced stage of her disease. A tunnelled intrathecal line was placed in the upper lumbar level and she was started on an infusion of hydromorphone and clonidine combination, which was gradually titrated up whilst withdrawing her subcutaneous diamorphine infusion. The patient was very well supported by her family as well as the community palliative care team, district nurses, as well as her own GP. The pre-filled syringe was prepared at the hospital pharmacy aseptic unit and was changed every week by the community palliative nurse. The holiday went well without any untoward incidents and the patient continued to survive for another 5 weeks. She died on the care of the dying pathway, which was instituted about 36 hours prior to her death. The family was supported by the community team.

Conclusion

This case illustrates the complex nature of the problems including pain in patients with pelvic malignancy. In addition to visceral and neuropathic pain, patients are often faced with autonomic disturbances. A good number of patients end up with urinary and faecal diversions, which give rise to body image and relationship issues and lead to low mood. Unless detected early and instituting curative treatment, the outcome of palliative treatment, although could prolong the life, would need a multidisciplinary approach for continuing care in a domiciliary setting.

The role of early pain interventions should be discussed with patients after counselling about rare, though potential, neurological and autonomic complications. Escalation of systemic opioids and addition of drugs like benzodiazepines and ketamine should be instituted only after careful consideration of their impact on quality of life due to unpleasant and undesirable side effects like constipation, drowsiness, and cognitive disturbances.

The role of intrathecal analgesia should be explored if this is available, with preference to an implantable system. Oncological treatments like radiotherapy and palliative chemotherapy as well as the use of bisphosphonates for bony metastases, can have a dramatic effect on pain in certain situations.

The roles of counselling and supportive care services are very important to ensure that the needs of the patient and their families are adequately met in these difficult situations.

Patients with advanced pelvic malignancy have complex problems that are often multifactorial and need a multidisciplinary approach. In addition to neuropathic and visceral pains, patients often have autonomic disturbances that affect the quality of life and independence. A multimodal patient-focused approach with emphasis on continuing supportive care is essential for optimal management of these patients.

Key learning points

- Pain during the early stages could be managed with simple analgesics, opioid titration, and adjuvant neuropathic agents.
- Oncological management not only helps with disease control, but also aids in pain management.
- Urinary and faecal diversion may be needed for symptom control.
- The role of interventional management with superior hypogastric plexus and ganglion impar blocks should be considered early.
- Advanced interventions like intrathecal infusion, cordotomy, and intrathecal neurolysis may be required for intractable pain based on expected survival, availability, and fitness.

Further reading

Başağan Moğol E, Türker G, Kelebek Girgin N, Uckunkaya N, Sahin S (2004). Blockade of ganglion impar through sacrococcygeal junction for cancer-related pelvic pain. Agri, **16**, 48–53.

Deer TR, Smith HS, Burton AW, Pope JE, Doleys DM, Levy RM, et al. (2011). Comprehensive consensus based guidelines on intrathecal drug delivery systems in the treatment of pain caused by cancer pain. Pain Physician, **14**, E283–E312.

Erdine S, Yucel A, Celik M, Talu GK (2003). Transdiscal approach for hypogastric plexus block. Reg Anesth Pain Med, **28**, 304–8.

Van den Beuken-van Everdingen MH, de Rijke JM, Kessels AG, Schouten HC, van Kleef M, Patijn J (2007). Prevalence of pain in patients with cancer: a systematic review of the past 40 years. Ann Oncol, **18**, 1437–49.

Mesothelioma and chest wall pain

Manohar Sharma and Sanjeeva Gupta

Introduction 70
Case discussion 71
　Background information 71
　History 71
　Pain description 71
　Medications 71
　Impact on daily living 71
　Other treatments for pain 72
　Investigations 72
　Scenario and expectations 72
Assessment and examination findings 73
　Relevant issues for management 73
Pain control options 74
　Relevance of pain relief option in current context 74
Treatment offered 76
　Outcome 76
　Follow up at 4 weeks 76
　Recurrence of pain after 6 months 76
　Management options 76
Conclusion 77
　Key learning points 77
Further reading 78

Introduction

Approximately 1800 new cases of mesothelioma are diagnosed each year in England. Most people who develop mesothelioma have worked in jobs where they inhaled asbestos, or were exposed to asbestos dust and fibres in other ways. The large majority of patients will die within a year of diagnosis. Mesothelioma incidence is still rising and is expected to peak between 2010 and 2015. Between 2006 and 2020 up to 30,000 people will die of the disease in the UK. Patients with mesothelioma frequently suffer distressing symptoms including breathlessness, chest pain, fatigue, and weight loss.

Intractable pain in particular is a key issue. Pain is caused by tumour compressing on the remaining lung, pleural effusion, and infiltration of tumour into chest wall and neural structures. Often the pain can be as a result of surgery to resect the tumour or take biopsy. Pain can often be controlled with simple analgesics and strong opioids in line with the WHO analgesic ladder. However, in a number of cases pain is refractory and severe. In these cases pain management options including nerve blocks, intrathecal neurolysis, spinal infusions, and cordotomy must be accessible and considered early.

Case discussion

Background information
The patient complained of severe right-sided chest wall pain for the last 3 months. He understood that he had incurable cancer. He had been treated with a combination of strong opioids and conventional analgesic and adjuvants, which initially helped. Of late his pain had become very debilitating. He had no other areas of pain apart from the right chest wall. He had well-controlled hypertension.

History
A 70-year-old man presented to his primary care physician with a history of increasing right chest wall pain and shortness of breath over a period of several months. Before retirement he was a shipyard worker. He was sent to the regional thoracic centre and was fully investigated. He had been diagnosed with malignant pleural mesothelioma. The tumour could not be safely resected or cured. He had pleural effusion and this was felt to be associated with shortness of breath. Drainage of pleural effusion had helped in improving shortness of breath. He was also suffering from progressive fatigue. The right-sided chest wall pain was becoming intolerable. He had been treated by his GP with a combination of various analgesics, which initially helped. He was referred to the local palliative care team and his medications were further escalated. He had been referred to the joint pain and palliative care clinic for assessment to see if he could be helped further with pain control. The oncologist felt that he was unsuitable for further chemo- or radiotherapy.

Pain description
He had constant pain. Pain was in most of the right chest wall. Pain was spontaneous and sharp and shooting at times. He scored pain 6–10/10 on brief pain inventory (BPI) as average pain. Pain was much worse (10/10 on BPI) with walking. Resting did not ease his pain.

Medications
His medications included: tablet morphine sulphate slow release 150mg twice daily, morphine sulfate solution 50mg 2-hourly as and when required (using four to six doses per day), gabapentin 1.2g three times daily, paracetamol 1.0g four times daily, diclofenac sodium 50mg three times daily, oral ketamine 50mg four times daily, and ramipril 10mg daily to control hypertension.

Impact on daily living
The patient initially had good pain control when his GP prescribed and titrated medications. Now the pain was waking him at night and some nights he was not able to sleep at all. He could not plan to go out as pain was mostly severe and disabling, though there was some reduction with current prescribed analgesics. He could not see the rest of his life living with this level of pain. Medications were making him tired, nauseous, constipated, and drowsy.

Other treatments for pain

The patient had tried transcutaneous electrical nerve stimulation (TENS), topical heat patch, lidocaine plasters and physiotherapy, but these had not helped his symptoms and he had stopped these (see Chapter 16).

Investigations

- Chest X-ray as shown in Figure 7.1.
- CT scan findings: right inferior chest wall infiltration with tumour along with significant pleural involvement. Tumour size significantly larger than previous scan 3 months ago.
- Biopsy result: epitheliod mesothelioma.
- Blood results: no abnormality

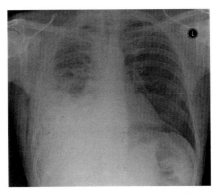

Figure 7.1 Chest X-ray showing involvement of right hemithorax with mesothelioma.

Scenario and expectations

- The patient attended the clinic with his family. He was in a lot of pain as evident from his history and from non-verbal clues regarding pain.
- He thought he was having an injection today and would go home afterwards. He had some information about cordotomy from community palliative care nurses.
- He was hoping to go on holiday next week.

Assessment and examination findings

Physical examination revealed retracted chest wall as in Figure 7.2, decreased breath sounds in the right lung base associated with dullness to percussion.

There was no neurological deficit or enhanced sensitivity on sensory examination of chest wall. There was no tenderness in thoracic spine.

He was able to hold a conversation without getting short of breath. He was able to lie supine for about 45 minutes. The rest of the parameters relating to examination (blood pressure (BP), heart rate, pulse oximeter oxygen saturation on room air) were within normal range.

His expected survival was about 6 months.

Relevant issues for management

- The patient had severe uncontrolled pain. He was on a total of 600mg oral morphine per day. He was getting sedative side effects from morphine. It was very unlikely that continuing to increase his morphine dose would improve his analgesia.
- He did not have an adequate understanding of pain control options. He needed admission to a hospice to control his symptoms and to enable discussion regarding further pain control options, when he was not as distressed.

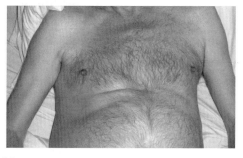

Figure 7.2 Showing retracted right chest wall as a result of mesothelioma.

Pain control options

1. Opioid rotation
2. Paravertebral and intercostal block
3. Intrathecal neurolysis
4. Continuous epidural/intrathecal analgesia by external pump
5. Intrathecal drug delivery system (IDDS)
6. Percutaneous cervical cordotomy.

Relevance of pain relief option in current context

1. Opioid rotation

Opioid rotation should be considered as a first-line option as his pain had not responded as well to dose escalation. It may that there is further local spread of tumour involving the rib cage and neural structures, making the pain much more severe. This option will be better considered as an inpatient admission to hospice. Opioids may also be delivered by syringe driver or topically (patch) and this can be more effective if there are doubts about absorption of orally administered opioids.

2. Paravertebral and intercostal block

Paravertebral and intercostal blocks are one of the options, but the pain relief may not be good as the pain distribution is in multiple dermatomes. At best the pain relief may last a week or two and at worst the patient may get a pneumothorax from the procedure. Continuous paravertebral infusion may have some benefits and efficacy but will need ongoing input from the treating team to manage the infusion logistics.

3. Intrathecal neurolysis

Intrathecal neurolysis is a very good option for pain control if the pain distribution involves one or two dermatomes. Intrathecal neurolysis in the thoracic region is much more difficult than in other parts of the spinal column (see Chapter 18).

4. Continuous epidural/intrathecal analgesia by external pump

Continuous epidural infusion may be effective to control pain in the patient. However, there will be a need to monitor this on a daily basis so as to review the analgesic epidural mixture and catheter site for any infection or catheter migration. This may also be an issue if there is no local support and governance to monitor safety of this treatment in the community setting.

5. Intrathecal drug delivery system (IDDS)

IDDSs can effectively deliver small doses of morphine and other analgesics directly into the CSF. This can achieve prompt pain relief, with much smaller doses of opioids than with the oral or parenteral routes. However, intrathecal infusion by implantable pump (reservoir) is generally considered effective for pain below the diaphragm, unless the intrathecal catheter tip is sited very close to the affected dermatome. There is some controversy regarding the safety of placing an intrathecal catheter in the mid thoracic region (see Chapter 12).

6. Percutaneous cervical cordotomy

Percutaneous cordotomy was considered a very good one-off option in this case (see Chapter 16). Open surgical cordotomy would not be an option in this case as the upper level of pain was at the T4 dermatome. Open cordotomy is effective for pain below the T6 dermatome. Percutaneous technique is much more common nowadays as the recovery period is much quicker and there is no morbidity that can be associated with open spinal surgical technique, which needs administration of general anaesthetic and the risks associated with general anaesthesia.

Treatment offered

The patient was admitted to the hospice on the same day. He underwent opioid rotation to OxyContin®. After 2 weeks he still had uncontrollable severe pain as at initial presentation. After further discussion with him and his family, he decided to undergo percutaneous cervical cordotomy. His opioids dose was reduced by half on the morning of cordotomy allowing him access to short-acting opioids. He tolerated the procedure well and had no pain immediately following cordotomy.

Outcome

He had further reduction in his opioid dose to about half as compared to initial oral morphine equivalent dose. He was able to go home without any chest wall pain.

Follow up at 4 weeks

The patient had no chest wall pain at 4 weeks after cordotomy. There was no change in his analgesic requirements. He was planning to go away on holiday.

Recurrence of pain after 6 months

The patient and his family got in touch with us after 6 months. They were able to go away on holiday to Europe for a week. Over the last few days, he had noted recurrence of pain and was feeling very tired and weak.

Management options

He was re-admitted to the hospice. He was assessed by the pain and palliative care team. He was terminally ill this time and was not expected to live more than a few weeks. He was not considered suitable for repeat cordotomy. Intrathecal neurolysis was not deemed to be safe and was not discussed. The option of tunnelled epidural catheter insertion or administration of opioids by syringe driver was discussed and explained to the patient and his family. A tunnelled epidural catheter was inserted in the mid thoracic region and this was connected to an infusion of morphine and levobupivacaine. This controlled his pain very well. He died 3 weeks later.

Conclusion

Key learning points

- Complex severe cancer pain patients must be assessed in an environment where there is close collaboration between the pain and the palliative care teams.
- Early referral should be encouraged for pain assessment of these patients. This did not happen in this case and the patient was on very high dosages of opioids.
- The patient may not need interventional pain technique at an earlier stage, but, early referral helps patients to understand the treatment options (including risks and benefits) and to develop a rapport with the treating team, in case the intervention was required at short notice.
- Pain assessment: it is very important to diagnose the characteristic of pain, i.e. neuropathic, nociceptive, or incident-type pain as this has relevance to the management plan.
- Informed consent is vital in these patients as cordotomy can have serious complications, though these are rare.
- Periprocedure care of these patients must be in an appropriate environment (trained staff skilled in looking after pre- and postcordotomy patients, opioid weaning-related issues, to deal with palliative care-related issues, i.e. fatigue, distress related to cancer, and poor prognosis, etc.).
- Cordotomy should not be offered as a salvage procedure or too late for the patient to tolerate and benefit from it. They should have a life expectancy of 6–12 months to derive optimum benefit from it.
- Cordotomy should only be offered to a patient who has a confirmed cancer diagnosis and poorly controlled pain despite treatment based on the conventional WHO analgesic ladder.

Further reading

Please also refer to chapters elsewhere in this book about cervical cordotomy (Chapter 16), intrathecal pumps (Chapter 12), neurosurgical techniques for pain relief (Chapter 20), and spinal neurolytic blocks (Chapter 21).

Bain E, Hugel H, Sharma M (2013). Percutaneous cervical cordotomy for the management of pain from cancer: a prospective review of 45 cases. *J Palliat Med*, **16**(8), 901–7.

Jackson MB, Pounder D, Price C, Matthews AW, Neville E (1999). Percutaneous cervical cordotomy for the control of pain in patients with pleural mesothelioma. *Thorax*, **54**, 238–41.

Mesothelioma Framework (2007). Available at: ℘ <http://www.mesothelioma.uk.com/editorimages/DOH%20Framework%20for%20Mesothelioma.pdf> (accessed 20 April 2013).

Price C, Pounder D, Jackson M, Rogers P, Neville E (2003). Respiratory function after unilateral percutaneous cervical cordotomy. *J Pain Symptom Manag*, **25**(5), 459–63.

Unilateral upper limb plexopathy pain caused by cancer

Andrew Jones

Introduction   *80*
Left breast carcinoma case discussion   *81*
Apical left lung carcinoma case discussion   *83*
Right apical lung carcinoma case discussion   *84*
Pain specialist's role in hospice settings   *85*
Conclusion   *87*
   Key learning points   *87*
Further reading   *88*

Introduction

This chapter explores the idea that while nerve blocks may have a place in the treatment of upper limb plexopathy, the interventional pain doctor must carefully assess all factors contributing to a patient's distress.

Three patients with cancer who had upper limb pain due to brachial plexus damage will be discussed. They each had different problems to consider in their management. These include separating pain from loss of function, fear about prognosis, and the future.

Left breast carcinoma case discussion

A 70-year-old woman, J, with left breast carcinoma was treated with simple mastectomy and radiotherapy. She presented at the interventional pain clinic complaining of left arm and hand pain. She also suffered from weakness and dysaesthesia of the hand. In addition, she had a phantom left breast but this caused no distress. On examination, she had wasting of the muscles of the hand and a glove distribution of numbness to touch and pin prick.

Although bothered by clumsiness of the left hand she was otherwise very active. During this episode I met her pushing her mother in a wheelchair.

J was very intolerant of medication and suffered severe drowsiness and dizziness with gabapentin, pregabalin, amitriptyline, and opioids. After discussion, the patient and I agreed on a trial of interventional techniques. These were performed as an outpatient at the hospice.

A brachial plexus block performed by axillary approach gave reasonable pain relief, but only for the duration of action of the local anaesthetic.

A stellate ganglion block was discussed. Informed consent was given although some consternation was caused by her remark that she hoped she did not suffer any complications as she was flying to watch her football team play in a Champions League match that evening. Fortunately the procedure was uneventful. However, pain relief was again only for the duration of action of the local anaesthetic.

A one-shot, high thoracic epidural injection produced the now familiar result of analgesia for the duration of action of the local anaesthetic.

The success of nerve blocks whilst the local anaesthetic was working suggested that long-term analgesia might be reliably achieved using continuous infusion of local anaesthetic via a catheter. However, as J was currently disease-free and could anticipate a long life span, the inconvenience of having to carry a pump and the risks of infection made this an unsatisfactory option. The patient understood that pain relief would not be accompanied by improvement in function of the hand. Clumsiness was a major part of her distress.

We agreed that she would learn to live with the disability and she expressed gratitude for my efforts. No further interventions were planned and she was discharged from the clinic.

I met J some years later when I provided local anaesthesia for her mother's cataract surgery. She remarked that her hand was much worse. I invited her to attend the hospice outpatient department again. On examination, the little and ring fingers of the left hand were clawed and the numbness was more pronounced in the ulnar distribution. Nerve conduction studies confirmed a peripheral ulnar nerve deficit superimposed on a brachial plexopathy. Ulnar decompression resulted in an improvement in symptoms. Understanding that her residual symptoms were due to brachial plexus damage from radiotherapy helped her coping strategies.

Our next meeting was to administer local anaesthesia for her own cataract surgery. J told me that she had had a recurrence of her carcinoma. Her hand symptoms of clumsiness had worsened, although pain was less of a feature. However, she did suffer from left shoulder pain. Examination revealed a tender glenohumeral joint and suprascapular nerve block gave long-term pain relief for this.

Our final meeting was some 10 years after our first when J was an inpatient in the hospice for drainage of ascites. She died 2 weeks later but had been to a football match the week before.

Apical left lung carcinoma case discussion

The patient, W, was a 76-year-old man who had an apical left lung carcinoma. This was causing pain and disability in his left shoulder, arm, and hand. The pain was controlled somewhat with the highest tolerable dose of pregabalin; the dose was limited by drowsiness. He felt that drowsiness was sufficiently troubling; he expressed enthusiasm for any intervention which might help the pain.

He suffered from ischaemic heart disease and was becoming increasingly short of breath which was also causing significant distress.

On examination he had numbness to touch and pin prick, but no hyperaesthesia or allodynia, in the medial aspect of the lower arm and hand. The shoulder revealed no glenohumeral tenderness but there was a trigger point in the trapezius.

The relative merits and complications of various interventions were discussed. Interscalene brachial plexus block was felt to have a good chance of improving his hand pain and perhaps shoulder pain. However, he was concerned by the risk of serious complications including intrathecal injection. Supraclavicular block carried a risk of pneumothorax in an already breathless man. In this situation the use of local anaesthetic and the risk of nerve damage could have made numbness and loss of function worse.

In view of the shoulder component of the pain a trigger point injection was performed.

When he returned for review, he felt that the trigger point injection had been ineffective. At that stage increasing numbness was distressing and he still felt that he wanted to explore interventional techniques for analgesia. Lateral cordotomy was discussed. It was emphasized that although this would very likely help with pain, it would have no effect on the numbness and clumsiness, but would at least not worsen it.

He was referred to a colleague who regularly performed cordotomy. After discussing the risks and benefits, W decided that the possible improvement in his symptoms did not justify the risks of the procedure, particularly in view of his comorbidities.

Right apical lung carcinoma case discussion

The patient, C, was a 63-year-old man with a right apical lung carcinoma. As well as involving the brachial plexus the tumour had encircled the subclavian vein. The tumour was resistant to oncological treatment and continuing to grow in spite of chemotherapy. At first referral, C was vigorously trying to be enrolled in a trial of a new chemotherapeutic regimen in another part of the country. Although pain was a feature of his brachial plexopathy, loss of function was his main problem He worked as a book-keeper and he could not now hold a pen. He was determined that if his symptoms were controlled he would be able to return to work. He was clearly very distressed by his diagnosis and poor prognosis.

Interventional techniques were discussed. On hearing that these would not improve his function and that they would not assist a return to work C declined any nerve block. He later travelled for consideration of taking part in the chemotherapy trial but was told he was not suitable. This had a devastating effect on him. He did not return for any further discussion of interventional techniques.

Pain specialist's role in hospice settings

The interventional pain specialist works as part of a multidisciplinary palliative care team. It is tempting to regard one's role as simply being a technician. However, the interventional doctor must have regard for all causes of the patient's suffering. The distress from pain must be rigorously differentiated from that caused by spiritual pain and from loss of function. Neither of these will be alleviated by nerve blocks and may be made worse.

The interventional doctor should be able to recognize spiritual pain, which is a part of the total pain described by Dame Cicely Saunders. Total pain is distress caused by a variety of negative feelings, which include pain, but also fear and anger. Loss of independence and hope for the future may also be features. Worry about what will become of family and dependents causes distress.

Spiritual pain is hard to define and may need arbitrary and personal meanings. Spirituality is common to all people and can include a sense of meaning, beliefs, and, for some, religion.

A doctor caring for a patient with any active disease should distinguish and try, as far as possible, to alleviate suffering. Suffering is distinct from physical symptoms and will not be relieved by technically satisfactory interventions. In fact, interventions have the capacity to increase suffering.

Suffering due to active cancer involves loss of personhood. A dualistic approach of mind and body discourages understanding of personhood and may cause more distress to the patient. The doctor may help with recovery from suffering by lending strength.

The interventional pain specialist should resist the understandable temptation to be a mere technician. Unfortunately colleagues in palliative care medicine may regard the interventionist as exactly that.

A survey of palliative care consultants in 2002 found that although all felt that the interventionist's role included advice on technical procedures, <25% felt that their role should extend to advice on prescribing analgesics.

While many patients will derive great benefit from interventional pain techniques, those whose suffering comes from spiritual or total pain will not. In fact, the pursuit of pain control with nerve blocks may worsen suffering. The patient may be given false hope of relief; intervention may distract from deeper analysis of the patient's distress; and the patient may lose faith in his doctors because they are so clearly missing the point.

Communication between members of the multidisciplinary team is important in focusing on the potential value of an intervention, but more important still is the team's communication with the patient. Multidisciplinary working can improve the individual's decision-making. The final decision remains with the patient.

The three patients described in this chapter all had pain as part of their suffering, but in each this was only a part. Attempts to control their pain by interventional techniques had no benefit in relieving distress.

Although C complained of pain, his extreme suffering was due to his lack of acceptance and fear of his advancing disease. His desperate search for an effective treatment and fixation on returning to work were both symptoms of profound spiritual pain. As soon as he discovered that interventional pain techniques were for symptom control and would have no effect on disease progression he showed little engagement with the interventional clinician. In particular, he was very upset by his inability to return to work as he could not hold a pen. His work had become a marker of progress for him. If he could work he must be getting better. His desperation to find a successful treatment stopped acceptance of his poor prognosis and caused much suffering. Rendering his arm and hand pain free would not have relieved his total pain. Referring for recruitment in a trial of chemotherapy and considering interventional pain techniques in fact exacerbated his severe total pain.

W showed much greater acceptance of his situation and was reluctant to undergo interventional techniques which had the risk of worsening other symptoms such as breathlessness and loss of function. In spite of side effects, he felt that his analgesic medicine gave good enough control of pain. Although he had several attendances to consider interventional options, each time he felt that the risks outweighed any possible benefit. In his case, loss of function was more of a problem than pain. He was accepting of his disease and prognosis. His general condition caused little suffering. Consequently, concern over making his other symptoms worse was uppermost in his mind.

J suffered distress from a loss of feeling of self. Although she was disease free, the treatment for her breast cancer had left her feeling that her body and her life were not as before. She experienced extreme frustration with the clumsiness of her left hand.

J was grateful for the attempts to improve her pain control with interventional techniques and seemed outwardly content. However, her mother once said 'J suffers terribly, you know'. The interventional techniques represented a possible missed opportunity to address spiritual pain.

When she re-attended after some years she was very frustrated by loss of function. The subsequent surgery to decompress the ulnar nerve did improve function and reduce distress. Also, we were able to talk more deeply about her feelings and the spiritual pain was partly addressed.

Her suffering eased after she had a recurrence of her cancer. It was as though, now that she was no longer disease free, she could accept feeling different to her former healthy state. For some weeks before her death she was in good spirits.

In conclusion, as well as skill in a variety of physical techniques the interventional pain doctor should bring empathy and understanding to the multidisciplinary team caring for a patient who needs palliation.

Conclusion

Key learning points

- Although nerve block may be seemingly indicated, the causes of distress should be carefully evaluated.
- Loss of function may be a more serious problem than pain, and will not be ameliorated by interventional techniques.
- The contribution of spiritual or total pain must be actively sought and assessed. Interventions may worsen spiritual pain.
- The interventional pain doctor should never be regarded as a simple technician.

Further reading

Cassell EJ (1982). The nature of suffering and the goals of medicine. *N Engl J Med*, **306**, 639–45.

Crawford GB, Price SD (2003). Team working: palliative care as a model of interdisciplinary practice. *Mes J Aust*, **179** (6), S32–S34.

Linklater GT, Long MEF, Tiernon EJJ, Lee MA, Chambers WA (2002). Pain management services in palliative care: a national survey. *Palliat Med*, **16**, 435–9.

MacLeod R (2007). *Total pain—physical, psychological and spiritual. Goodfellow Symposium, 2007.* Available at: ℅ <http://www.fmhs.auckland.ac.nz/soph/centres/goodfellow/_docs/total_pain_handout.pdf> (accessed 20 April 2013).

Diffuse cancer pain in lower half of body

Kate Marley

Case discussion 90
  Introduction 90
  History 90
  Pain 90
Admission to hospice and pain management 91
  Ketamine 91
Cancer and pain progression 92
Repeat admission to hospice and total pain 93
  Methadone 93
  Total pain 94
  Epidural analgesia 94
Further pain management options 96
  What are the further management options for pain? 96
  Intrathecal drug delivery 96
  Intrathecal pump implantation 97
Conclusion 99
  Key learning points 99
Further reading 100

Case discussion

Introduction

Here we will consider a complex case of refractory pain in a patient with advanced cancer which illustrates the challenges of balancing benefits and burdens of different treatment strategies. This case highlights the advantages of collaboration between pain medicine, palliative care, oncology, and neurosurgical teams to achieve the most favourable outcome for the patient.

History

- The patient was a 69-year-old lady who had been undergoing treatment for metastatic breast cancer for 6 years.
- Two years ago, she was seen in the palliative medicine outpatient clinic and complained of pain in her back, right hip, and right leg.
- She was known to have disease in her lumbar vertebrae, para-aortic lymph nodes, and also a soft tissue mass in her pelvis.
- She had been treated with several different chemotherapeutic agents over the years.

Pain

- The pain in her back, right hip, and right leg had some neuropathic features (burning and shooting) although the patient found it difficult to describe it fully.
- It was worse on movement but also present at rest.
- It seemed to be only partially responsive to strong opioids and was severe despite up-titration of oxycodone MR (OxyContin®) tablets to 160mg twice daily.
- She had developed side effects with various neuropathic agents and was not able to tolerate more than 150mg pregabalin twice daily.

The pain has several causative factors: bony pain from the lumbar disease, neuropathic and visceral pains from the pelvic mass and lymphadenopathy. It may not be fully responsive to opioids and other approaches may be needed.

What could be done next to manage the pain?

Admission to hospice and pain management

The patient was initially reluctant to consider admission to the hospice as she had witnessed several patients dying during her previous admissions to the oncology centre and this had started her thinking about her own mortality. She saw admission to a hospice as 'giving in to the inevitable' and 'the beginning of the end.' However the pain was so severe and was limiting her everyday activities that she agreed to be admitted for a short period of time.

During her admission to the hospice 'burst' ketamine was administered by CSCI for a few days with good effect on the pain. She was discharged home after this course was complete to be seen in clinic within 2 weeks.

Unfortunately at her next palliative medicine outpatient appointment the pain was starting to recur and in view of the good response to subcutaneous ketamine, oral ketamine 10mg three times daily was started. Two weeks later she was reviewed and the pain was improving but not controlled so the ketamine was up-titrated to 20mg three times daily. Alongside these changes OxyContin® dose was reduced to 120mg twice daily.

Ketamine

- Ketamine is a potent NMDA receptor-channel blocker which is used for pain difficult to control with standard analgesics. It can be given via the oral, sublingual, subcutaneous, or intravenous routes.
- The 'burst' regimen used initially in this case involved using ketamine 100mg over 24 hours in a syringe driver with the dose gradually increased to 300mg then to 500mg over 24 hours CSCI over a period of 5 days at which point it was stopped. Using this sort of regimen, improved pain control may persist for several weeks after the treatment for some people. This procedure can be repeated as required. Midazolam or haloperidol is used alongside the ketamine to prevent the dissociative symptoms sometimes associated with it.
- Oral ketamine may also be used where pain persists beyond the 'burst' regime. Liaison between the patient's general practitioner and community pharmacist is required to ensure the patient does not run out of ketamine as the oral preparation is obtained by special order.
- With long-term use there may be a risk of urinary tract problems such as cystitis.

The patient found that her pain was stable for 6 months and she was able to continue with oncological treatments and carry out normal activities of daily living during this time. She was not completely pain-free but episodes of pain were less intense and more responsive to OxyNorm® IR liquid.

Cancer and pain progression

After 6 months the same pain started to recur with increasing intensity until it dominated her life and prevented her from going out with her husband at weekends. A recent CT scan had shown progression of the cancer in the lymph nodes and pelvis.

What could be done next?

What other information would be helpful in managing this lady's pain?

She was very distressed by both the pain and recent news of disease progression. She had discussed further chemotherapy with her oncologist and had mixed feelings about this. Her last round of chemotherapy had been exhausting and she had had a traumatic episode in hospital with neutropenic sepsis. On the one hand she was dreading the thought of further chemotherapy and on the other she saw it as her only chance to live.

Her oncologist had been very concerned about her pain and subsequent reduction in functional ability and had suggested to her that a further admission to the hospice might be helpful. Her palliative medicine consultant shared this opinion. She felt that she had no choice but to go back into the hospice. She had faith in the team at the hospice as they had helped her pain before. She also felt she could talk to the team in the hospice about her hopes and fears regarding her illness.

Repeat admission to hospice and total pain

The patient had previously told the consultant and other team members in the hospice about her feelings about the cancer and this continued during this admission. She was a devout Christian and prayed to God to give her strength to overcome her illness initially and then when it became clear that the illness was incurable, she prayed for the strength to withstand the treatments and for more time to spend with her family.

She described feelings of anger about the cancer appearing at this time in her life and feeling 'cheated' out of the retirement she had planned with her husband. They had planned to travel to make up for holidays not taken when they were building their business and in particular they had wanted to visit their daughters in Spain and Japan.

At times she found herself questioning her faith and this was especially distressing for her. The vicar at her church had been extremely supportive of the patient and her husband and she felt reluctant to confide in him as she didn't want to 'let him down.' However she talked these spiritual issues through with the hospice chaplain which she found very helpful, and was eventually able to disclose her feelings to her vicar who was as supportive as ever.

In conjunction with the psychological and spiritual support she received in the hospice, her analgesic regimen was significantly modified. The ketamine was increased with some effect and a decision was made to convert to methadone using the Morley–Makin method of titration.

On admission to the hospice she was taking:
- Ketamine 30mg three times a day
- OxyContin® MR 140mg twice a day
- Pregabalin 150mg twice a day
- OxyNorm® IR liquid 40mg prn.

On discharge from the hospice she was taking:
- Ketamine 50mg three times daily
- Methadone 45mg twice a day and 15mg prn
- Pregabalin 150mg twice a day
- OxyNorm® IR liquid 60mg prn.

Methadone
- The strong opioid was rotated to methadone in the hope that it would result in improved pain control for this lady.
- Methadone titration is not straightforward and is done in the inpatient setting in the majority of cases in palliative care because the patient must be observed closely for signs of toxicity.
- The regimen used in this case was described by Morley and Makin and involves stopping the regular strong opioid and then titrating methadone over several days before converting to a regular, twice daily dose.

Total pain
- Alongside the titration of the analgesia, our patient was allowed to voice her concerns about her illness and the effect that it was having on her life and on those close to her.
- The concept of 'total pain' was described by Dame Cicely Saunders and emphasizes the psychological, spiritual, and social dimensions of pain.
- She was distressed by the loss of her retirement, had started to question her faith, and felt anger about what was happening to her and by having the opportunity to articulate those concerns she was then able to address them with help as needed.

The patient found the methadone very helpful for the pain initially and continued as an outpatient for a further 6 months. However the pain increased in intensity, especially the pain down her right leg. She developed a right foot drop and her palliative medicine consultant ordered an MRI spine which was reported as showing:

'Extensive infiltration of the sacrum and disease within L2 and L5. Metastases are not causing any significant spinal canal narrowing and appearances of the spinal cord and cauda equina are satisfactory. It is possible that the sacral infiltration is causing some neural tissue compression.'

Having the MRI scan was extremely painful and she was unable to lie flat for any length of time. Radiotherapy was desirable as a treatment for the pain. However in order to receive this treatment, she would need to be able to lie flat. She was devastated at yet more bad news with regard to her disease and readily agreed to hospice admission to optimize her pain in order to undergo radiotherapy.

What modifications could be made to the analgesic regimen now?

Epidural analgesia
Up-titration of methadone did not help the pain and the palliative medicine consultant asked for an opinion regarding epidural analgesia from the consultant in anaesthesia and chronic pain management who worked in collaboration with the hospice team.

An epidural was sited with infusion containing diamorphine, clonidine, and levobupivacaine. The methadone was weaned off completely during this time.

Pain control improved and she was able to lie flat. She was therefore transferred to the regional oncology centre for five fractions of radiotherapy to the lumbar spine and sacrum with the epidural *in situ*. Plans were made for return to the hospice for refilling of the epidural pump should this run out during her stay in the centre.

The patient was then transferred back to the hospice for further rehabilitation and pain control. The epidural had to be replaced due to leakage and pain remained problematic with escalating doses of diamorphine in the epidural.

One month later the epidural was delivering 85mg diamorphine per day along with levobupivacaine and clonidine. The epidural catheter became disconnected and she soon developed a fever. She had no new neurological signs and an urgent MRI of her spine did not reveal any evidence of an abscess.

The epidural was removed and she was given alfentanil infusion 40mg over 24 hours via a syringe driver.

Further pain management options

What are the further management options for pain?

1. Re-titrate strong opioids. The reason an epidural was tried was because opioids by conventional routes were only partially effective for her pain so this may not be viewed as the most favourable option.
2. Resite the epidural. This is not without problems. It would mean frequent visits from district nurses at home and the risks of disconnection and infection will remain. However, she had felt more benefit from epidural analgesia than with oral opioids.
3. Intrathecal pump delivering analgesia. The patient could not access this option locally and would have to be referred into a tertiary centre. There would still be a risk of infection and the 'incident' component of the pain may not be helped by this method of delivery of analgesia.
4. Cervical or open cordotomy for right leg pain.

The patient and her doctors discussed the options and she decided that she wanted to find out more about having an intrathecal pump device. Her consultant referred her to be seen jointly by a consultant in chronic pain management and a palliative medicine consultant in outpatients at another hospice.

In clinic the options for analgesia were discussed with the patient and her husband and when discussing the risks and benefits of an intrathecal pump she was told that she could realistically expect that the pain control could be improved at rest. There would be a significant risk of infection and the pump would not improve the foot drop or increase her mobility.

Intrathecal drug delivery

Collaboration between the pain medicine and the palliative care service enabled selection of the most appropriate procedure for the patient and enabled her to make a fully informed decision about the pump.

This was presented as an option to this lady because of the complex nature of her pain. There was no single neuroablative procedure that was likely to help her and she had had complications with epidural analgesia. Oral and subcutaneous analgesia were not improving her pain control and she was suffering more side effects as doses escalated. Intrathecal delivery of opioids produces good analgesic response in relatively small doses with few systemic side effects.

With improved analgesia it was hoped that she would be more comfortable at rest and that with better pain control she might be able to move around more although this was by no means a guarantee, particularly as her mobility was limited due to the foot drop.

It was hoped she would be able to spend more time at home given that the pump is internal and it would not need to be refilled so frequently.

Intrathecal pump implantation

The patient decided to go for an intrathecal pump and was therefore admitted to the tertiary neurosurgical centre for a trial of intrathecal bolus analgesia containing morphine 1mg and bupivacaine 2.5mg. She found this beneficial and plans were made for the intrathecal device to be implanted 1 week later.

Her medications on admission were as follows:
- Alfentanil 40mg 24 hours CSCI
- Levomepromazine 12.5mg 24 hours CSCI.

She underwent implantation of an intrathecal infusion pump into the left side of her abdomen. The pump used was a Synchromed II with a 40mL reservoir. The initial doses of intrathecal medication were:
- Morphine 1.5mg per day
- Bupivacaine 5mg per day.

She suffered some drowsiness initially. The alfentanil in the syringe driver had been reduced at implantation of the pump to 20mg and then very quickly was reduced to 10mg then 5mg over 24 hours, stopping completely within 48 hours of the procedure.

The medications in the pump were adjusted to:
- Morphine 2.8041mg per day
- Bupivacaine 9.3747mg per day.

Pain control was significantly better and she was discharged back to the hospice for ongoing care. She made good progress with rehabilitation and managed to get home for Christmas with her family.

> Once again the patient was discharged back to the hospice from the regional centre to undergo discharge planning. She needed to have a further reassessment from the physiotherapist and the occupational therapist in view of the change in her pain control to evaluate any improvement in level of independence and consider what equipment would help her at home.

After Christmas she underwent a staging CT scan and saw her oncologist. The news was not good and the CT now showed:
- Nodules at right and left lung bases
- Right hydronephrosis. Ureter dilated to iliac vessels where there was a 5x3.4cm soft tissue mass involving the iliac artery and vein
- Para-aortic nodes had increased in size
- New right iliac nodes
- Sclerotic changes right iliac crest, sacrum, L2, and L5.

The pain started again to increase in her back and right hip and further chemotherapy was planned. A peripherally inserted central catheter line was inserted in anticipation of this. Some palliative radiotherapy was planned prior to starting the chemotherapy to attempt to control the pain coming from the right iliac blade.

Unfortunately when she attended for the radiotherapy she was unable to lie flat due to the pain and even with breakthrough analgesia was not able to tolerate the scan required for radiotherapy planning. The pain did not respond to an increase in the dosage of intrathecal drugs and so transfer back to the neurosurgical ward was arranged.

She was seen by the pain medicine, palliative care, and neurosurgical teams daily. With up-titration of the intrathecal medications and coordination of breakthrough analgesia and lorazepam prior to each session, she was able to have her daily radiotherapy sessions at the local oncology unit whilst an inpatient on the neurosurgical ward.

She was transferred back to the hospice for ongoing symptom management and psychological and spiritual support.

The strength of the medications in the pump on discharge was:
- Morphine 25.78mg per day
- Bupivacaine 45.118mg per day.

The dosage remained the same and her pain remained under reasonable control until her death some months later.

Conclusion

Key learning points
- Cancer pain is complex and multifactorial in origin, multiple treatment modalities are likely to be needed to manage it.
- Collaborative working between pain medicine, palliative care, neurosurgical, and oncology services is needed in such cases.
- Intrathecal delivery of opioids and local anaesthetic can be effective for managing complex pains refractory to oral analgesia.
- It is important to address the psychological, spiritual, and social dimensions of pain alongside the management of the physical symptoms.

Further reading

British Pain Society (2008). *Intrathecal Drug Delivery for the Management of Pain and Spasticity in Adults: Recommendations for Best Clinical Practice*. Available at: ℘ <http://www.britishpainsociety.org/itdd_main.pdf> (accessed 20 April 2013).

Clark D (1999). 'Total pain', disciplinary power and the body in the work of Cicely Saunders, 1958–1967. *Soc Sci Med*, **49**, 727–36.

Fallon M, Welsh J (1996). The role of ketamine in pain control. *Eur J Palliat Care*, **3**, 143–6.

Jackson K, Ashby M, Martin P, Pisasale M, Brumley D, Hayes B (2001). 'Burst' ketamine for refractory cancer pain: an open-label audit of 39 patients. *J Pain Sympt Manag*, **22**, 834–42.

Morley JS, Makin MK (1998). The use of methadone in cancer pain poorly responsive to other opioids. *Pain Rev*, **5**, 51–8.

Storr TM, Quibell R (2009). Can ketamine prescribed for pain cause damage to the urinary tract? *Palliat Med*, **23**, 670–2.

Upper gastrointestinal pain from invasive pancreatic cancer

Matthew K. Makin

Case discussion *102*
  Initial assessment *102*
  Further assessment *102*
  Pain presentation and assessment *102*
  Cancer diagnosis and surgery *103*
  Recurrence of pain and initial management *103*
  Cancer recurrence and further management *104*
Pain escalation and management in hospice settings *105*
  Surgery for pain control *105*
  Pain recurrence *106*
  Pain related to cancer metastasis and management *106*
Conclusion *108*
  Key learning points *108*
Further reading *109*

Case discussion

The patient is a 56-year-old lady who presented as an emergency with a 7-day history of jaundice, dark urine, pale stools, and itching skin. There was no history of pain preceding her attendance to her GP, but she thought she may have unintentionally lost about 3kg or 4kg in weight. She was a health-care worker who had no risk factors for liver disease; she did not drink alcohol and was not taking any regular medication; of note her brother had died of carcinoma of the pancreas before his 60th birthday.

Initial assessment

- On first assessment and on examination the patient was noted to be deeply jaundiced with fullness palpable in the right upper quadrant. There were no stigmata of chronic liver disease.
- Blood tests showed an elevated serum bilirubin at 207 µmol/L and other liver function tests were deranged with alanine aminotransferase (ALT) 712 units/L and alkaline phosphatase (ALP) 685 units/L.

Further assessment

- She was initially investigated with an ultrasound scan of her abdomen; no discrete lesions were identified during this examination, either within the liver or in the head of the pancreas. The sonographer reported that the patient's common bile duct was dilated at 14mm.
- She went on to have imaging with CT of chest, abdomen, and pelvis 3 days after her initial assessment. The CT was suggestive of biliary obstruction that was traceable down to a stricture in the distal common bile duct.
- In view of the suspicion of bile duct pathology she went on to have endoscopic retrograde cholangio-pancreatography (ERCP). The images at the time of examination were consistent with cholangiocarcinoma. Brushings were taken for cytology and an intraluminal stent was deployed to resolve the biliary obstruction.

Pain presentation and assessment

The day after this procedure was when the patient first reported pain:

- The pain was well documented as being a constant, upper abdominal 'ache' radiating through to the back and exacerbated by lying on the left side.
- The pain scored 9/10 on a VAS with the pain scoring 5/10 at its least intense.
- On examination there was tenderness in the upper abdomen, the patient was tachycardic, restless, and unwell.
- Blood tests showed an elevated serum amylase of 2400 units/L suggesting a diagnosis of postprocedure pancreatitis.

The patient remained on the surgical unit and she was assessed by the hospital acute pain team who advised using intravenous patient-controlled analgesia (PCA), and although she only used a minimal amount of morphine (10mg over 24 hours) this proved to be most effective. Consensus at this time was that the clinical and radiological diagnosis was cholangiocarcinoma (tumour marker tests were unhelpful; cancer antigen (CA)

19.9 was elevated at 54 units/mL, carcinoembryonic antigen (CEA) 15 units/mL, CA-125 67 units/mL). The PCA was only required for 48 hours and the postprocedure pancreatitis, and the associated pain syndrome resolved spontaneously over a period of 72 hours.

Cancer diagnosis and surgery

Cytology brushing from the ERCP confirmed the diagnosis of cholangiocarcinoma. The case was discussed at the local upper gastrointestinal (GI) cancer team meeting and the patient was referred to the regional hepatobiliary centre for assessment. She underwent major surgery (a pylorus-preserving pancreato-duodenectomy). Postoperative histology confirmed the diagnosis of a moderately differentiated adenocarcinoma in keeping with primary cholangiocarcinoma with lymph node involvement. Pathological staging was pT3pN2 (Figure 10.1). The surgical procedure took place 5 weeks after her original presentation. She was well for 10 months following surgery but then developed steadily increasing upper abdominal and back pain. At this time her functional status was good (performance status 1).

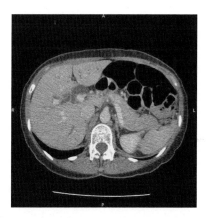

Figure 10.1 Showing minimal disease around coeliac plexus.

Recurrence of pain and initial management

The patient presented to her GP with upper abdominal and back pain that she described as being persistent and aching in nature, the pain disturbed her sleep at night. The pain was rated as 7/10 at its worst and 3/10 at its least. The discomfort was exacerbated by lying flat and only partially relieved by intermittent doses of co-codamol, 30/500mg.

Her medication was adjusted in primary care, and pain was partially controlled with a combination of ibuprofen 400mg three times a day, co-codamol 30/500mg, 2–4-hourly prn, and tramadol MR 100mg twice a day. During the day the pain did not interfere with her functional status significantly, but there were still episodes when it hurt sufficiently to disturb her sleep.

Cancer recurrence and further management

A restaging CT scan showed an area of soft tissue in the region of the coeliac plexus (Figure 10.2), and a clinical and radiological diagnosis was made of recurrent disease 14 months after the initial presentation. She was referred to the oncology team to consider palliative chemotherapy; however, she declined the offer of treatment as on balance she felt the chance of benefit was outweighed by the probability of intolerable side effects.

Co-codamol and tramadol were discontinued and her pain was managed with a therapeutic trial of MR morphine 30mg twice a day and intermittent doses of IR morphine 10mg as required 2–4-hourly. On a typical day she required between four to five additional doses of analgesia. Unfortunately this did not give an acceptable balance between side effects and analgesia, and therapy was complicated by dysphoria, sedation, and intermittent hallucinations and visual misperceptions. Morphine was discontinued and MR oxycodone was used in its place. The dose of oxycodone MR escalated to 50mg twice a day with 20mg of IR oxycodone as required.

This did reduce the pain intensity at night to between VAS 2–3/10 that allowed the patient to sleep, or return to sleep following a dose of oxycodone IR. During the day there were episodes when the patient reported being pain free. The situation was further improved by the judicious introduction of a small dose of gabapentin as an adjuvant analgesic initially at 100mg at night but the dose was titrated up in 3-day intervals with steady increments to a total dose of 300mg three times a day.

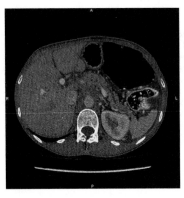

Figure 10.2 Showing disease around coeliac plexus.

Pain escalation and management in hospice settings

Sadly this improvement was not maintained, the pain syndrome escalated and she was referred to see the specialist palliative care service. The patient was despondent and exhausted by the discomfort, and felt she was losing faith in the medication and in the health professionals that had been supporting her. Interestingly the pain syndrome was typical of that seen in patients with advanced carcinoma of the head of the pancreas; namely a gnawing relentless pain that is particularly severe when lying flat, with an associated epigastric discomfort, and an affective element.

Sleep at night was disrupted; the patient was locked into a cycle of pain, insomnia, exhaustion, and despondency. Pain was only partially responsive to combinations of strong opioid, adjuvant, and non-opioid medication, and the trajectory of escalation was upwards, at what appeared to be an exponential rate. Dose-limiting side effects prohibited further escalation of opioid and adjuvant analgesia.

Surgery for pain control

The patient had lost a further 10kg in weight, there was nothing, however, of significance to find on abdominal examination other than the surgical scars; neurological and sensory testing examination was unremarkable. At this time the differential diagnosis was either radicular spinal pain and/or potential spinal cord compression. Given the CT findings, however, the clinical and radiological diagnosis that underpinned the pain syndrome was thought to be recurrent cholangiocarcinoma with infiltration into the coeliac plexus. Following this diagnosis an early referral was made to consider a bilateral intrathoracic splanchnicectomy (BITS procedure) and the patient was assessed by the upper GI laparoscopic surgeon, following agreement of this approach by the multidisciplinary team (MDT).

There was some initial uncertainty about whether this procedure would offer a good outcome to the patient as it is a method that, although is documented to work well in patients with pancreatic pathology, it remains unproven and doubtful whether it would benefit patients with pain syndromes that were not caused directly by cancer of the pancreas. In view of the nature of the symptoms, however, it was agreed to proceed with the procedure on a trial basis. She underwent the BITS procedure a month after the assessment by the specialist palliative care team. The procedure took place under general anaesthetic and involved full pleural division bilaterally, as well as division of all splanchnic nerves anteriorly from T4 to the costodiaphragmatic recess. Only a matter of hours after recovery it was apparent she had an excellent analgesic response to the procedure. The dose of OxyContin® MR was titrated down to only 10mg twice a day, the dose of gabapentin was also titrated down over the following month; however, she remained on gabapentin 300mg at night, as she found this dose had an excellent hypnotic effect.

On review in clinic pain was under good control (VAS 2/10 at worst, 0/10 at least), her sleep was not disturbed, she felt less exhausted, and psychologically more robust. Functional status improved, however the one complicating factor that caused the patient new and additional distress was frequent, malodorous, pale loose bowel motions that occurred between four to six times a day; these were not relieved by a therapeutic dose of Creon®. The diarrhoea was investigated by colonoscopy which revealed some diffuse thickening of the large bowel from the rectum down to the caecum. Following completion of antibiotic therapy her condition stabilized.

She declined chemotherapy and a repeat CT 6 months after her previous imaging showed very little progression in the soft tissue lesion in and around the coeliac plexus. Pain at this time was still under good control, with sleep pattern, appetite, and mood being no cause for concern.

Pain recurrence

- A month later she developed intermittent episodes of colicky abdominal pain, and bloating associated with borborygmi and nausea.
- She presented as an emergency with abdominal distension, vomiting, and severe abdominal pain.
- X-ray and CT demonstrated sigmoid volvulus and she underwent a limited hemicolectomy and ileostomy.

Following her surgery however, she seemed to gain less benefit from taking MR OxyContin®, but appeared to benefit disproportionately when taking IR oxycodone. This is probably related to the fast transit time to her ileostomy despite taking a combination of Creon®, codeine phosphate, and loperamide.

The worrying ongoing symptom for 2–3 months following the treatment of the volvulus was ongoing diarrhoea with symptoms suggestive of malabsorption. She was referred to the GI and dietetic team 2 months after the procedure. The diarrhoea was diagnosed as being secondary to malabsorption as a complication of bacterial overgrowth, and treated with a course of broad-spectrum antibiotics. She was treated for bacterial overgrowth with Augmentin® and indeed the frequency of her diarrhoea appeared to settle following this. She was stable for the month following this and indeed the local surgical team considered reversal of her stoma.

Regrettably, a restaging CT scan before the reversal showed ascites and evidence of peritoneal disease as well as new small volume metastases in the right lobe of the liver. Taking these into consideration it was agreed that reversal of the stoma would be inappropriate.

Pain related to cancer metastasis and management

- Twenty-four months following the initial diagnosis she presented with new hip pain that escalated rapidly over a 2–3-week duration.
- The pain was episodic in nature, associated with weight bearing and scored VAS 9/10 at worst and 2/10 at its least.
- On examination there was severe pain on internal rotation of the right hip and plain film showed a destructive lesion in the right pubic ramus and acetabulum (Figure 10.3).
- The dose of OxyContin® MR was escalated to 50mg twice a day.
- Unfortunately the lesion was neither suitable for radiotherapy nor orthopaedic surgical intervention.

- In view of the intractable pain she was referred for, she underwent a percutaneous spinothalamic cervical cordotomy.
- That gave a partial relief of symptoms, and although the intensity of pain decreased to VAS 4/10, the dose of OxyContin® MR remained unchanged and the patient required between four to six doses of OxyContin® IR on a daily basis.

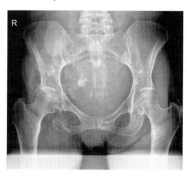

Figure 10.3 Showing destructive lesion around right pubic ramus and acetabulum.

Unfortunately her functional status deteriorated significantly over a number of weeks and she was admitted to a local hospice for terminal care. When it was not possible to give medication via the oral route, in the last days of life, symptoms were controlled by using diamorphine 80mg and clonazepam 2mg given as a CSCI over 24 hours.

Conclusion

Key learning points

- Close collaboration between disease-specific speciality, oncology, palliative care, and pain medicine is vital to offer appropriate diagnostics and range of pain control options.
- Pain can be related to many causes and accurate diagnosis and assessment of the type of pain is important to offer appropriate treatment options.
- Surgical techniques targeting the removal of cancer pain pathways may be more effective than pharmacological management alone.
- Coeliac plexus block has a good evidence base for pain control and reducing the need for opioids in pain related to pancreatic cancer, and thereby improving quality of life.

Further reading

Arcidiacono PG, Calori G, Carrara S, McNicol ED, Testoni PA (2011). Celiac plexus block for pancreatic cancer pain in adults. *Cochrane Database Syst Rev*, **16**(3), CD007519. Available at: <http://onlinelibrary.wiley.com/doi/10.1002/14651858.CD007519.pub2/pdf> (accessed 21 April 2013).

Yan BM, Myers RP (2007). Neurolytic celiac plexus block for pain control in unresectable pancreatic cancer. *Am J Gastroenterol*, **102**, 430–8.

Multiple bone metastasis-related incident pain

Manohar Sharma

Incident pain *112*
 Introduction *112*
 Bone metastasis-related incident pain *112*
 Spinal instability-related incident pain *113*
Case discussion *114*
 Referral information *114*
 Pain description *114*
 Impact on daily living *114*
 Medications *114*
 Investigations *114*
 Clinical scenario and patient's expectations *115*
 Assessment *115*
 Examination findings *115*
 Relevant issues for management *115*
Pain control options *117*
 Pain relief options in current context *117*
 Treatment offered *117*
 Other issues in perioperative period *118*
 Outcome *118*
Complications *119*
 Follow up at 4 weeks in referring hospice *119*
Patient feedback in relation to cordotomy *120*
Conclusion *121*
 Key learning points *121*
Further reading *122*

Incident pain

Introduction

This chapter will focus on one very complex and difficult to manage cancer pain. Incident pain is the pain brought about by movement and is usually related to pathological fracture of long bones. Incident-type pain may also result from spinal metastases leading on to spinal instability. These patients may then be very difficult to nurse, especially if they also have spinal cord compression-related motor weakness. Usually patients have very little pain at rest and the slightest movement causes very severe pain. Incident pain responds poorly to opioids. Epidural and intrathecal infusions need to include local anaesthetic in analgesic mixtures in high doses to control pain, but this can cause numbness and other side effects related to sympathetic blocking actions of local anaesthetics on spinal cord. Incident pain responds well to treatment directed at treating the cause of pain, e.g. surgical fixation of long bone pathological fractures, spinal fixation if there is spinal instability, or cordotomy if the pain is focal and unilateral.

Bone metastasis-related incident pain

A common cause of incident pain is bony metastasis which is usually caused by prostate, breast, and lung cancer. Pathological fractures can cause severe movement-related pain (incident pain). Usually these pains are better controlled by surgical fixation of the fracture site. However, in some cases, if there is poor fixation of pathological fracture because of extensive local metastatic disease, the incident pain can become difficult to control with the usual WHO analgesic ladder-based approach. An example of this type of pathology causing pain is shown in Figure 11.1.

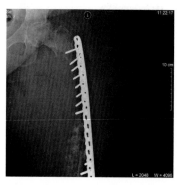

Figure 11.1 Despite extensive surgical fixation, this patient has severe incident pain making nursing care and mobilization nearly impossible.

Spinal instability-related incident pain

Another cause of incident pain is from secondaries to spine. These can cause spinal cord compression and also the pain caused by spinal instability. It is very important in these cases to recognize the pain pattern and obtain spinal surgical opinion about spinal fixation or stabilization. Figures 11.2 and 11.3 show examples of a patient who had severe incident pain as described and was on very high dosages of opioids, but pain was well controlled after spinal fixation.

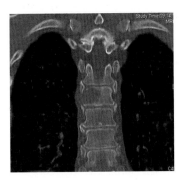

Figure 11.2 This patient had severe incident pain which was poorly controlled with high opioid dosages.

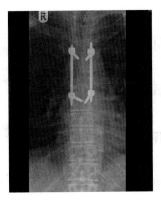

Figure 11.3 Same patient as in Figure 11.2 whose pain was well controlled after spinal fixation.

Case discussion

The patient was 56 years of age and had been diagnosed with osteochondrosarcoma affecting her right pelvis. She had been referred to the author's unit to control severe pain in her right leg. She had this pain for nearly 6 months. Tumour had infiltrated the area of her right pelvis and had eroded through the neck of femur and was now also infiltrating her right sciatic nerve. She had been reviewed by her GP, local palliative care team, local orthopaedic team, oncologist, and local chronic pain team. She was advised by the orthopaedic team to undergo amputation of her right leg, but this was felt to be too extreme a treatment option by her. She wanted to explore other treatment options. She had local radiotherapy and chemotherapy and more was not an option.

Referral information

This patient was referred from out of the region from the author's hospital. It was about 5 hours' drive by an ambulance. She had osteochondrosarcoma affecting her right pelvis and now involving right sciatic nerve. The local pain clinic and palliative care did not have the facilities to control the pain further. She was an inpatient at a local hospice. This patient was given an expected survival of about 4 months, though this was 12 months ago.

Pain description

She had moderate spontaneous pain at rest. On brief pain inventory this was scored as 5/10. However, on slight movement in her right leg, her pain became excruciating (10/10), making it very difficult for her to roll or turn in bed. Pain was sharp, stabbing, and very intense on movement.

Impact on daily living

She was wheelchair bound because of inability to stand and walk. Turning in bed was very painful. She was comfortable at rest with the current analgesic regimen. She was on many analgesics and these made her drowsy, but did not control her pain. Her appetite was poor.

Medications

These included: OxyContin® 600mg twice daily, OxyNorm® 140mg 4-hourly, pregabalin 150mg twice daily, amitriptyline 100mg at night, regular paracetamol, diclofenac, senna, and lansoprazole.

Investigations

CT scan of her pelvis as seen in Figure 11.4, sent from her hospital showed fracture involving right neck of femur, pubic ramus, and acetabulum. Her other blood tests were normal. She was found to have lung metastases, but these did not compromise her breathing at rest.

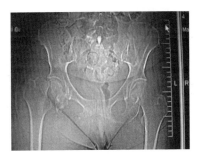

Figure 11.4 CT scan image showing fracture through right neck of femur, missing pubic ramus on the right side.

Clinical scenario and patient's expectations

- The patient had been sent for consideration of cordotomy.
- The patient was very keen to go on a holiday, once the pain was well controlled.
- The patient was expecting to reduce opioid dose significantly, i.e. more than half of the current dose, because of side effects.

Assessment

She was assessed jointly by pain and palliative care consultants following admission to the author's hospital. She was tired and drowsy because of lack of sleep and medications. She was very anxious and distressed as pain was very poorly controlled. She found any slight movement involving her right leg to be excruciating and was unable to manage standing. Her pain was mainly of incident type (on movement only). She was expected to live for about 6 months. She was desperate to undergo any suitable procedure if she was suitable. She was not short of breath and could lie supine for about 45 minutes without any difficulties.

Examination findings

- Very distressed because of right groin and leg pain
- Overweight
- Right leg externally rotated
- No sensory loss in right lower limb
- No autonomic features of temperature, colour change, or swelling
- Motor weakness, but difficult to assess because of pain
- Managing to mobilize in wheelchair if right leg was kept immobile
- Severe pain on any movement of right leg
- Good respiratory reserve as assessed by simple bedside tests for respiration.

Relevant issues for management

- She had incident pain and partially controlled spontaneous background pain.
- Her mobility including any movement of right leg was restricted.
- Her sleep was impaired because of poorly controlled incident type pain.

- She had difficulty with self-care and needed help.
- Her appetite was poor.
- She was drowsy.
- Wished to go for holiday and spend quality time with her partner.
- Her quality of life was very low because of cancer but also as a result of poorly controlled pain and side effects of high dosages of various analgesics.
- Consenting a patient for a major pain relief procedure with potentially serious though rare complications was an issue to be aware of. This was managed by discussion of the procedure with the patient and family a number of times, offering the patient information leaflet regarding the procedure, and admitting the patient a day before the procedure to allay any concerns.

Pain control options

1. Intrathecal drug delivery (ITDD) system
2. Continuous epidural/intrathecal analgesia by external pump
3. Percutaneous cervical cordotomy
4. Open surgical cordotomy.

Pain relief options in current context

1. Intrathecal drug delivery system

ITDD systems can effectively deliver morphine and other analgesics directly into the CSF. This can achieve prompt pain relief, with much smaller doses of opioids than with the oral or parenteral routes. In our patient, this option was not considered for two main reasons: firstly, the patient had been referred from out of our area, and her local pain service could not provide support for the device, particularly pump refills. The second reason was that intrathecal infusion may not control the incident type pain well, but may be effective for background spontaneous pain. See Chapter 17.

2. Continuous epidural/intrathecal analgesia by external pump

The absence of local logistical support also made continuous tunnelled epidural impossible. Intrathecal pump and epidural infusion can be helpful in diffuse pain in the lower half of body, but their efficacy in incident pain is not well established. One will need to infuse sufficient dosages of local anaesthetic in the infusion mixture which, in turn, will cause numbness and weakness in lower limb. See Chapters 12 and 17, and the cordotomy section (Chapter 16).

3 and 4. Percutaneous cervical cordotomy and open surgical cordotomy

Percutaneous and open cordotomy were considered to be equally suitable in this case. Percutaneous technique is much more common nowadays as the recovery period is quicker and there is no morbidity associated with open spinal surgical technique. In patients who may not be able to cooperate or tolerate percutaneous cervical cordotomy (cannot lie supine because of pain, very anxious to undergo cordotomy while awake), open surgical cordotomy is an alternative. Bilateral open cordotomy can be carried out in cases with complex, medically refractory cancer pain involving the lower half of the body. There is a much higher chance of sphincter control impairment, but this may not be an issue in a patient with very severe cancer pain who may otherwise be terminally ill. See Chapter 16.

Treatment offered

The patient underwent percutaneous cervical cordotomy. It was difficult to get her across the operating table because of severe pain she had in her right leg, especially on movement. She tolerated the procedure well and had no pain immediately following cordotomy. Transfer across onto the bed from the operating table did not produce any pain. Opioid dose was reduced by half on the morning of cordotomy allowing her access to short-acting opioids, if needed.

Other issues in perioperative period

In the recovery area, the patient was noted to be very anxious, tachycardic, restless, and had no pain in her right leg. When asked, she was not able to tell what the problem was. She was very agitated. What could be the problem?

On reviewing her drug card, it was noted that her dose of OxyContin® was reduced from 600mg to 300mg on the morning of cordotomy. However, there was some error on the ward and she was only given 30mg OxyContin®. Immediately diagnosis of opioid withdrawal was made and she was administered intravenous fentanyl as it was immediately available in the recovery area and further oral dose of OxyContin®. This immediately settled her symptoms.

Outcome

Next day she had no pain in her right leg, but complained of very slight pain in similar location in her left leg. She did not have this pain before. This new pain in her left leg settled after 2 days. She also complained of neck stiffness and headache for a couple of days after the procedure. Her mobility improved and she now could walk with the help of a frame as compared to being in a wheelchair. Her dose of OxyContin® was reduced to 150mg twice a day at the time of discharge from the hospital 5 days after cordotomy. She had managed to come off pregabalin, amitriptyline, and OxyNorm® at the time of discharge.

Complications

The patient had neck stiffness and headaches for 2 days after cordotomy. She also felt general malaise which is very common post cervical cordotomy. This is related to the response to a major neuroablative procedure and to significant reduction of opioid dose.

She developed very mild mirror pain (pain in left leg in similar location as in right leg) in left leg the day after the procedure. This settled very soon. In rare circumstances mirror pain can become as severe as original presenting pain.

She developed burns on her fingers after she fell asleep with a cigarette in her hand. However, these were not painful because of the effect of cordotomy.

Follow up at 4 weeks in referring hospice

She attended 4 weeks after the procedure at her local hospice. Her pain was very well controlled and the plan was to further wean her opioids. She was planning to go away on holiday in Europe, which she did. She died 6 months after the cordotomy and had pain relief lasting until her death.

Patient feedback in relation to cordotomy

The patient and referring physician were delighted with the response to cordotomy and the extent of pain control. The patient found the procedure somewhat difficult, but thought that it was worth undergoing.

Conclusion

Key learning points

- Complex severe cancer pain patients must be assessed in an environment where there is close collaboration between pain and palliative care teams.
- Early referral to specialist team should be encouraged for pain assessment, if pain is becoming difficult to control. This did not happen in this case and the patient was on very high dosages of opioids and other analgesics.
- The patient may not need interventional pain technique at earlier stage, but this helps the patient to understand the treatment options (including risks and benefits) and to develop rapport with the treating team. This is relevant in case the intervention was required at short notice.
- Pain assessment: it is very important to diagnose the characteristic of pain, i.e. neuropathic, nociceptive, or incident type pain as this has relevance to management plan (incident pain responds poorly to opioids).
- Informed consent is vital in these patients as cordotomy can have serious complications, though these are rare.
- Periprocedure care of these patients must be in appropriate environment (trained staff skilled in looking after pre- and postcordotomy patients, opioid weaning-related issues, to deal with palliative care-related issues, i.e. fatigue, distress related to cancer, and poor prognosis, etc.).
- Opioid management in perioperative period is critical. The patient may become opioid toxic from excellent pain control from cordotomy. This patient suffered opioid withdrawal because of nursing issues on the ward.
- Cordotomy should not be offered as salvage procedure or too late for the patient to tolerate and benefit from it. They should have life expectancy of 6–12 months to derive optimum benefit from it.
- Cordotomy should only be offered to patients who have confirmed cancer diagnosis and poorly controlled pain despite treatment based on conventional WHO analgesic ladder.
- Despite good pain control, these patients often require significant and ongoing support from the palliative care team and for this reason the importance of close collaboration between the teams cannot be overemphasized.

Further reading

Please see chapters elsewhere in this book for cervical cordotomy (Chapter 16), intrathecal pumps (Chapters 12 and 17), neurosurgical techniques for pain relief (Chapter 20), and spinal neurolysis (Chapter 18).

Crul B, Laura BM, van Egmond J, van Dongen RTM (2005). The present role of percutaneous cervical cordotomy for the treatment of cancer pain. *J Headache Pain*, **6**, 24–9.

Jackson MB, Pounder D, Price C, Matthews AW, E. Neville (1999). Percutaneous cervical cordotomy for the control of pain in patients with pleural mesothelioma. *Thorax*, **54**, 238–41.

Lipton S (1968). Percutaneous electrical cordotomy in relief of intractable pain. *BMJ*, **2**, 210–12.

Lipton S (1973). Pain control and the management of advanced malignant disease. *Proc R Soc Med*, **66**, 7–9.

Chapter 12

Intrathecal pump for cancer pain

Louise Lynch

Case discussion 124
Pain clinic assessment and management 125
   Pain clinic assessment 125
   Initial management 125
   Intrathecal test dose 125
Intrathecal pump 127
   Pump implantation 127
   'Pump not working' 127
   Exploration and revision of IT pump 128
   Bacteraemia and meningism following pump revision 128
   Medtronic analysis report of the explanted pump 129
   Reimplant of intrathecal pump 130
   Loss of pump efficacy 130
   Current condition 131
Conclusion 132
   Key learning points 132
Further reading 133

Case discussion

The patient was referred to the pain clinic with a history of worsening perineal and left leg pain and lack of response and side effects with strong opioids. She had a long history of left leg pain, having had both a femoral fracture and excision of an osteoid osteoma at the age of 6. She had been under review by the orthopaedic surgeons and had last seen them 5 years previously for an opinion regarding a stiff left hip. This pain was well controlled at the time and was described as more of 'a stiffness' than pain.

The patient was first referred to the gynaecologists with a 6-month history of a lump in her perineum. This was thought to be a benign cyst, but the histology report after excision came back as 'a spindle cell tumour approximately 4x4x4cm, surface ulceration with, microscopically a moderate to severe degree of cytological atypia'—a leiomyosarcoma.

The patient was referred to oncology for adjuvant brachytherapy and had placement of 12 needles interstitial radioactive implants to the tumour bed. Nine needles were actually used after CT planning and she went on to receive 30 Gy in six fractions at two fractions/day. Local pain as a result of the 'expected radiation reaction' was managed with MST® (slow-release morphine) 20mg twice a day and morphine sulfate solution 10mg 4–6-hourly.

Unfortunately, the patient went on to develop a more severe radiation reaction than expected and at the end of the brachytherapy was complaining of severe vaginal pain, described as 'burning', 'throbbing', and 'unbearable spasms'. A pelvic MRI scan performed at the time showed no obvious cause for this and no evidence of tumour recurrence. Slow release morphine was restarted at a dose of 10mg twice daily.

At the next few oncology appointments it was clear that pain was worsening and as there was felt to be a neuropathic element (sharp, stabbing, spontaneous) to it, the patient was commenced on pregabalin—initially at a dose of 50mg twice a day but titrating up to three times a day, and then 100mg three times daily. The patient continued with the slow release morphine at a dose of 10mg twice daily. The possibility of referral for a 'nerve block' was discussed. The patient's pain was recorded as well managed on this regimen.

The patient then went on to develop radiation necrosis of her perineum and presented acutely with painful ulcers shortly after her radiation reaction pain was recorded as well controlled. At this point the slow release morphine was increased to 20mg twice a day, the pregabalin was increased to 200mg three times a day and the co-codamol changed to morphine sulfate solution 10mg as required. A psychology referral was arranged.

The patient's perineal pain was documented as well controlled on the further addition of fentanyl patch 75 micrograms/hour with paracetamol 1g four times daily and ibuprofen 600mg three times daily. However, a new problem was then described, which could have been due to pressure on the left sciatic nerve (S1 component) somewhere along its course. The pain described was sharp and lancinating in nature and spread from buttock to ankle. The pain was associated with frequent disabling episodes of leg giving way and with leg swelling. Straight leg raising was reduced to 45° on the left compared with 70° on the right.

Pain clinic assessment and management

Pain clinic assessment

At this point the patient was referred to our pain clinic with increasing perineal and leg pain even on strong opioids and with side effects (drowsiness) limiting the option of increasing the opioid further.

The working diagnosis was of possible left S1 sciatica together with perineal pain secondary to radiation damage. The concern was that the patient had recurrence of her perineal leiomyosarcoma and had sciatic compression somewhere on the course of the nerve through the pelvis. Neurophysiology was, however, reported as normal and an MRI scan performed 1 month later revealed degenerative changes at L3/4, L4/5 and L5/S1 with some osteophyte protrusion into spinal canal. There was no compromise of the spinal canal and no evidence of metastatic disease or pelvic insufficiency fractures.

There was no definite evidence of cancer recurrence at this stage, but her progressive symptoms still strongly suggested that this might ultimately prove to be the case.

Initial management

Initially she was offered caudal epidural steroid injection and this was repeated a further three times over the next year. The first injection was effective for 3 months, but this result was not sustained. Neither ganglion impar blocks nor hypogastric plexus blocks were helpful. A variety of medications including lacosamide, lamotrigine, and ketamine were tried and OxyContin® and OxyNorm® were substituted for fentanyl without much improvement in pain control.

Physiotherapy was initially very successful in that previously wasted muscle groups improved in bulk mass, strength, and control, but ultimately pain progressed to involve all of the left leg with associated tingling. The patient was finding it increasingly difficult to manage at home and at work and becoming increasingly distressed with her situation.

A further MRI scan was performed and showed degenerative changes as previously, but the presumed diagnosis was of tumour recurrence, although there was no definitive evidence of this. ITDD was an option and so the patient was listed for an intrathecal test dose and referred to the specialist pain nurses for an information session on ITDD systems.

Cordotomy was not considered to be an option as life expectancy was thought to be much greater than 2 years and spinal cord stimulation was not considered to be an option because of the need for repetitive MRI scanning to monitor disease progression. Since this decision was made, MRI-compatible spinal cord stimulation systems have become available.

Intrathecal test dose

- The patient had an IT test dose under X-ray screening because of high body mass index (BMI).
- 0.5mg hydromorphone was injected at L2/3 via a 24-gauge Sprotte needle. (The patient was taking approximately 100mg/day of oxycodone, equivalent to approximately 200mg/day of oral morphine.

If 200mg oral morphine is approximately equivalent to 1mg of IT hydromorphone, then a 12-hour test dose is approximately 0.5mg.)
- Other options would have been to add clonidine 15–30 micrograms and/or bupivacaine 1–2mg to the test dose if the hydromorphone had not produced a good effect.
- If the patient had proven recurrence and progression of the leiomyosarcoma then it may have been more appropriate to opt for a drug combination test dose.
- The test dose produced excellent result in terms of pain relief, which lasted for >24 hours.

Intrathecal pump

Pump implantation

- The pump was implanted and the procedure was performed under heavy sedation and local anaesthesia.
- Routine antibiotic cover at that time was a single dose of 1g intravenous flucloxacillin and 2mg/kg of gentamicin.
- The dural puncture was made at L2/3 via a paramedian approach under X-ray screening and the catheter tip sited at the upper border of T12.
- The pump was filled with 80mg of hydromorphone to a total of 40mL with water for injection (WFI).
- A priming bolus together with an additional 0.3mg was given via the pump in theatre; the background infusion rate was set at 1.0mg of hydromorphone/day.
- The 0.3mg bolus was chosen as 0.5mg had produced prolonged hypotension and the background infusion dose of 1mg was chosen, as this was the dose calculated from her oral opioid consumption.
- For cancer patients who have or may have progressive or recurrent disease, it is good practice to review them for pump refills and assessments every 4 or 5 weeks.
- So the mix was chosen to contain 2mg/mL hydromorphone in 40mL, which would last for at least 4–5 weeks allowing for doubling the background infusion if this became necessary.

Immediately postoperatively the OxyContin® halved to 20mg twice daily, the OxyNorm® and pregabalin doses were unchanged. The patient's postoperative course was uneventful and she was transferred back to her regular oncology ward after 16 hours and went home on the 3rd post-operative day.

On review 2 weeks later the patient still had some pain, but was happy with the level of pain relief. She had managed to stop OxyContin® and OxyNorm® and arranged a phased return to work. We increased the background infusion rate to 1.2mg hydromorphone/day and advised on a gradual reduction of pregabalin.

'Pump not working'

- Four months later a telephone call indicated a significant deterioration in pain control back to pre-pump levels. The patient had increased her pregabalin up to 100mg twice daily and her OxyNorm® up to 10mg four times a day.
- She was listed for a pump review under fluoroscopic screening.
- First, the pump was interrogated and the reservoir contents aspirated. The calculated reservoir volume should have been 14.9mL, but 40mL was aspirated.
- Pump malfunction or catheter occlusion was suspected.
- Second, the pump side port was accessed under X-ray screening. It was possible neither to aspirate CSF, nor to flush the catheter.
- The pump was refilled and set to a minimum background rate of 0.2mg/day of hydromorphone.
- The patient was advised to continue her current medication and listed for formal exploration and revision of the catheter and/or the pump.

Exploration and revision of IT pump

- The exploration and revision took place 1 month later under local anaesthesia and sedation and antibiotic cover.
- First, the catheter was reviewed. It was anticipated that the catheter would be occluded, but on disconnection of the catheter from the pump, CSF flowed freely from the end of it. Saline was injected easily into the catheter too. The catheter was not blocked.
- Catheter tip position was checked and was as previously, i.e. lying posteriorly in the spinal canal and at the upper border of the vertebral body of T12.
- Second, pump function was checked. The pump was programmed to deliver a single bolus of 0.5mL over 30 minutes (maximum flow deliverable by the pump is 1mL/hour) and sequential X-rays of the pump were compared to look for movement of the rotor arm. (The pump was, of course, disconnected from the patient at this point.) Rotor arm movement was clearly visible when sequential X-ray images were compared.
- No obvious problem was identified, but pump malfunction seemed the most likely culprit, even though rotor arm movement had been clearly seen and it is not a common problem.
- The pump was explanted and sent back to Medtronic for analysis. A new device filled with 80mg hydromorphone in 40mL WFI was implanted and a priming bolus with an additional single bolus of 0.3mg hydromorphone given. The background rate was set at 1.2mg/day.

Bacteraemia and meningism following pump revision

- The following day the patient started to complain of headache and nausea with retrosternal chest pain and became progressively unwell over the course of the day.
- Eventually medical staff were alerted urgently with a history of pyrexia, tachycardia, dropping conscious level (Glasgow Coma Scale (GCS) score of 10/15), meningism, hypoxia, and wheezing. The working diagnoses were of meningitis after pump revision and aspiration pneumonitis.
- An infection screen was performed including lumbar puncture after head CT to exclude raised intracranial pressure or cerebral event. Intravenous flucloxacillin and ceftazidime were administered on advice from microbiology.
- A few hours later the GCS score had improved to 15/15, although on initial assessment it was actually 14/15 rather than 10/15. Signs and symptoms of meningism persisted. The patient needed oxygen with a flow of >10 litres of O_2/minute to keep pulse oximetry readings >95%.
- CSF analysis was reported as 'Gram stain negative; glucose normal, but high white cell count and protein levels'.

The patient was transferred to the care of the infectious diseases team. The working diagnosis was of meningitis secondary to pump revision and either the pump or the catheter was the presumed source of the infection. There was a recommendation to remove the pump and catheter as the source of the meningitis.

Blood cultures isolated *Streptococcus oralis* and *Streptococcus mitis*—these are normal oral flora.

Chest X-rays had shown bilateral basal consolidation and bilateral hilar lymphadenopathy.

There was debate as to whether the streptococci had originated from the pump, catheter, skin, or from the oral cavity via aspiration.

The patient was managed with an initial 2-week course of intravenous ceftriaxone 4g once a day, which necessitated central venous access.

Clinically the patient improved quickly, although was still suffering from episodic headaches. Pain was well controlled.

The catheter was later removed leaving the pump *in situ*. There was a risk of colonization of the catheter whether or not it was the original source of the bacteraemia and thus a risk of recurrence of infection when the antibiotic course came to an end. Ultimately the risk was too great to leave it in place. The catheter was sent for culture as were swabs from the pump and pump pocket. All samples were negative apart from an incidental *Streptococcus faecalis* from a skin wound swab. The pump was filled with saline and left to infuse at a minimal rate.

Medtronic analysis report of the explanted pump

Analysis summary

The pump showed acceptable catheter access port testing, telemetry response, and alarm function. A review of the interrogation report did not reveal any anomalies; there were not any motor stalls to explain the large drug reservoir volume discrepancy. The drug reservoir was empty. The pump passed the 'Dispense Accuracy Tests'; the dispense accuracy (actual dispense versus programmed dispense) was within specification (±14.5%).

Conclusions

The pump passed infusion testing with no anomalies found. Since the catheter was not returned for analysis it remains inconclusive as to what could have been the root cause of the reported drug reservoir volume discrepancy.

Note

In similar reported events, analysis of the catheter revealed a misalignment of the catheter to the pump. This resulted in a drug reservoir volume discrepancy caused by occlusion.

The patient was under regular review by the infectious diseases team and at one point was reassessed by another consultant who had no previous knowledge of her and who noted severe dental caries. The consultant speculated that this could well have been the site of origin of the bacteraemia. The patient was referred to the dental hospital and underwent six extractions and three restorations.

The patient was without pain relief from the IT pump for 8 months, as it was felt to be wise to wait for 3 months after the dental extractions. The initial concern that the patient's severe pain was related to recurrence of her leiomyosarcoma seemed to be unsubstantiated and monitoring scans had all proved negative. Pain during this 8-month period was managed with pre-pump medication of OxyContin®, OxyNorm®, and pregabalin, although the patient's pain was by no means well controlled.

Reimplant of intrathecal pump

- The catheter was reimplanted under antibiotic cover as advised by microbiology.
- The procedure was performed entirely under local anaesthesia without sedation after the respiratory problems presumed secondary to aspiration after the last revision.
- Swabs were taken from the pump and pump pocket and sent for culture to microbiology.
- The first dural puncture was made at L1/2, but it was not possible to pass the catheter without excessive discomfort.
- A dural puncture was then made at L2/3 and a bolus of 2mL 0.5% bupivacaine given via the catheter at T9 for anaesthesia for exploration of the pump pocket in the right iliac fossa.
- The catheter was then withdrawn as far as the upper border of T12 as previously.
- The pump was emptied and refilled with 80mg hydromorphone and 1.2mg clonidine in 40mL WFI. (Clonidine was added because of its effect on neuropathic pain and the suggestion that it may protect against granuloma formation.)
- A priming bolus with an additional 0.3mg hydromorphone was given in theatre and the background infusion rate set at 1.0mg hydromorphone/ day.
- The pump was refilled 2 months later, but this time with 160mg hydromorphone and 1.2mg clonidine. The patient was complaining of an increase in her pain following a road traffic collision a couple of weeks previously so the background infusion rate was increased to 1.2mg/day.

Loss of pump efficacy

- The patient called to say that her pain relief was again suboptimal.
- At clinic review a week later it was clear that increasing the background rate had made no substantial impact on the patient's pain (performed a week ago). The options were then either to continue to increase the background infusion rate further, to change to a bolus-based regimen with a low background rate, or to alter the drug combination or to change the base drug.
- The problem with the first approach of continually increasing the opioid infusion is that tolerance can develop and the opioid infusion rate can start to increase significantly with a potential risk of dural granuloma formation to add to continual loss of clinical effect.
- The second option of reducing the background rate and using a bolus-based regimen is more elegant in that the patient is in complete control of their pain relief and uses drug only when necessary. This both gives excellent pain control and may theoretically reduce the chance of granuloma formation.
- The third option of changing the drug mix might well be helpful. Clonidine is effective in relieving neuropathic pain and may be helpful in reducing the risk of granuloma formation. The dose the patient was currently on was very low and could be increased—this might both improve the quality of pain relief and prove to be opioid sparing.

The addition of bupivacaine was another option and if the patient had progressive tumour it might be appropriate to add it at this stage. However, the working diagnosis was of a sciatic nerve injury secondary to radiotherapy and so there was not such an urgency to control the pain because of limited life expectancy.

- The fourth option was of changing the primary drug from hydromorphone to another opioid, or from opioid to clonidine, bupivacaine, or ziconotide.
- The patient had not reached the point where this would be appropriate, but there was an argument for the use of ziconotide if the current mix of hydromorphone and clonidine was unsuccessful.
- The decision was made to go with a low-background bolus-based regimen and to then to increase the clonidine in the mix if changing the mode of administration was not sufficient.
- The background infusion rate was decreased to 0.5mg/day and a bolus of 0.3mg over 5 minutes with a lockout interval of 10 minutes and a maximum activity of six per day was programmed to be administered via a patient therapy manager (PTM).

The patient attended again a couple of weeks later for a refill with the same mix of hydromorphone and clonidine. She reported some loss of efficacy of the 0.3mg bolus—still effective but lasting for only 3 hours rather than 6 hours as previously. A single bolus of 0.5mg was given via the single bolus function of the programmer and when this was confirmed to be effective without prohibitive side effects, the pump was reprogrammed to increase the PTM bolus to 0.5mg with the other settings as before.

The pump was filled with 160mg of hydromorphone and 2.4mg of clonidine to 40mL with WFI. Settings were otherwise unchanged.

The next refill 2 months later was with 160mg hydromorphone and 4.8mg of clonidine.

Current condition

- Last review indicated that the patient's pain was now well controlled and she had started a phased exercise programme and lost a substantial amount of weight.
- She was in full-time employment and was taking no additional oral analgesics.
- There was no evidence that her leiomyosarcoma had recurred and she had been discharged from routine follow-up by her oncology team.
- If the patient runs in to pain control problems in the future the next option would be to increase the dose of clonidine further.

Conclusion

Key learning points
- There are a number of choices of analgesic interventions for patients with cancer-related pain. The likely life expectancy of the patient, site of the pain, cause of the pain, and likely tumour progression are relevant factors to consider. If the patient has pain in a hemi-quadrant, as this patient, cordotomy might be appropriate if life expectancy is < 1 year, or neurolytic blocks if death is more imminent.
- There are a number of options for both intrathecal test doses and infusions. First, second, and third choice options should be planned.
- Managing 'pump not working' problems.
- Managing infection.
- Managing loss of efficacy of chosen drug mix and doses.

Further reading

Please see Chapter 17.

British Pain Society (2008). *Intrathecal Drug Delivery for the Management of Pain and Spasticity in Adults: Recommendations for Best Clinical Practice*. Available at: ℘ <http://www.britishpainsociety.org/itdd_main.pdf> (accessed 20 April 2013).

Deer TR, Prager J, Levy R, Rathmell J, Buchser E, Burton A, *et al*. (2012). Polyanalgesic Consensus Conference (2012): recommendations for the management of pain by intrathecal (intraspinal) drug delivery: report of an interdisciplinary expert panel. *Neuromodulation*, **15**, 436–66.

Hester J, Sykes N, Peat S (2012). *Interventional Pain Control in Cancer Pain Management* (see chapters 5–7). Oxford: Oxford University Press.

Details of interventional techniques

13	Basic procedure safety and patient considerations for cancer pain interventions	137
14	Sympathectomy for cancer pain	147
15	Vertebroplasty and kyphoplasty in spinal metastasis pain	167
16	Cervical cordotomy for cancer pain	181
17	Intrathecal drug delivery for cancer pain	197
18	Spinal neurolysis	227
19	Trigeminal interventions for head and neck cancer pain	239
20	Neurosurgical techniques for cancer pain	251
21	Peripheral nerve blocks including neurolytic blocks	263

Chapter 13

Basic procedure safety and patient considerations for cancer pain interventions

Samyadev Datta

History and physical examination *138*
  Introduction *138*
  Patient history *138*
  Investigations *138*
  Documentation *138*
  Algorithmic approach to interventions in cancer pain
    management *139*
Patient consent and expectations *140*
  Informed consent *140*
  Informed consent and informed refusal *140*
  Surrogate decision-making *140*
  Patient expectations *140*
  Patient preparation *140*
  Patient position *141*
Intervention support *142*
  Radiology technicians *142*
  Timeout *142*
  Assistance *142*
Intervention procedure *143*
  Procedure *143*
  During the procedure *143*
  Postprocedure care *143*
Conclusion *144*
  Key learning points *144*
Further reading *145*

History and physical examination

Introduction

Interventional procedures are an integral part of the options available for treatment of certain cancer-related pain. Well-trained physicians can use these techniques safely to provide patients with significant and long-lasting pain relief. Inclusion of interventional pain management options in the treatment plan should be based on the best available evidence for efficacy and safety based on the diagnosis and individual patient.

Patient history

Before any intervention is undertaken, it is mandatory to obtain a complete history and perform a physical examination. Cancer patients are known to complain of multiple pain processes, so it is necessary to identify the most painful site. Cancer patients with chronic pain may need the pain process that is causing the most limitation in function to be addressed first. Terminally ill patients would rather have the most painful issue addressed. An experienced physician will keep this in mind during the initial interview.

Investigations

As we decide to undertake any interventional procedure, we must review all relevant investigations. If there are any new symptoms or exacerbations of existing symptoms, consider new or additional investigations. If any spinal procedure is planned, please evaluate images of the spinal cord.

An expansible lesion on the head of the rib may cause severe radiating pain. Extension of the lesion into the thoracic outlet will also cause the same symptoms, and extension into the spinal cord may produce similar symptoms. Interventional approaches to these situations may be quite different. Intercostal neurolysis may be an option for a limited pain distribution not affecting any motor nerve roots.

A spinal cord stimulator may be an option for brachial plexopathy. Spinal opioids may also be considered. Space-occupying lesions in the spinal canal are associated with higher risk and morbidity, but it may be possible to thread a catheter above the lesion and potentially provide sufficient pain relief. Patients need to be educated about significant associated risks.

Compression fracture of the vertebra may cause significant axial pain. It may also result in radiating pain; therefore, these patients are amenable to treatment by vertebral augmentation. In the presence of metastatic lytic lesions in thoracic or lumbar vertebrae, another option is RFA of the tumour followed by vertebral augmentation.

Documentation

It is important to clearly document the plan for each patient. Documentation should include: the site, side of the body, and the intended procedure. This will be very helpful, since the planned procedure may not take place immediately after the physical examination. Documentation is especially important when a team of physicians is involved. In addition, some patients do complain of multiple pain processes, and on the day of procedure they may report that pain is at a different site. A review of the history and documentation will help to clarify the situation. Occasionally it may be necessary to re-evaluate and modify the procedure based on patient comments before the procedure.

Algorithmic approach to interventions in cancer pain management

When considering any intervention in cancer patients, using algorithms will allow you to approach any situation with assurance that the options are safe and appropriate. Use of evidence-based medicine should be considered in the decision-making. It is important to note that not all procedures have randomized controlled trials to provide strong evidence. Using good clinical judgement and best available evidence allow decisions to be validated. Experienced operators may also have a lot of experience in this field and feel comfortable to proceed, even though some procedures may be associated with high risk.

An example is the use of neurolytic saddle block for treatment of perineal pain in rectal carcinoma. A major risk associated with this procedure is incontinence of bladder and bowel. Discussion with the patient and family clearly identifying the risk may allow the patient to appreciate the potential benefits of the procedure. Intrathecal thoracic neurolysis at a single level for a rib metastasis is very useful, with low risk.

Patient consent and expectations

Informed consent

The importance of this document cannot be overemphasized. Interventional procedures, especially with neurolytic agents may be associated with significant risk and morbidity. Patients and their families must be educated on the risks. A well-informed discussion must be undertaken so that expectations of patients, families, and caregivers are clearly defined. Informed consent needs to be realistic. Informing a dying patient that one of the risks of procedure is death is meaningless. But on the other hand expecting that an intervention will reduce the pain load, and possibly reduction in medications and associated side effects is realistic. Very sick patients may not be in a position to understand or sign consent. Working with the patient's health-care proxy is an option.

Informed consent and informed refusal

As physicians and caregivers, we occasionally come across as condescending or overaggressive. We project the image that we know better. Our knowledge of diseases and treatment options gives us the advantage of being able to provide informed options to patients. The dilemma for us is that patients may refuse these choices. We must be prepared to accept the same, as it is the patient that we have to serve. We must maintain patients' autonomy.

Surrogate decision-making

As we have made great strides in medical care, we have also made advances in surrogate decision-making. Sometimes surrogates, with the best intentions, can be very aggressive, but as caregivers we must be ready to say no.

Our goal is to do our best, but occasionally we may need to step back and reassess the whole situation from all perspectives.

Patient expectations

This section demands clarification. Patients always want to have no pain after any procedure, so it is very important that the clinician set expectations before the procedure. Be realistic and explain clearly—raising expectations can be disappointing for all parties. Also, it must be clear that no two patients are alike and therefore may respond differently. Warning patients about complications is part of an informed consent, but expectations need to be addressed separately.

Patient preparation

Many of these patients will be very frail and in ill health. As caregivers, we need to be aware that just the process of transportation from room to procedure unit may be a great imposition on patients. Every effort needs to be taken to keep these to a minimum, done as carefully and efficiently as possible.

These patients may be dehydrated and nauseous. It is a good idea to have intravenous access and ensure adequate hydration. If they need medication to control any of their symptoms, be prepared. During the actual procedure they may need sedation. Medications used for sedation need to be administered incrementally to prevent any sudden change in vital signs.

Patient position

Most interventional procedures are done with the patient in the prone position. Occasionally patients may not be able to lie prone, so be prepared to be flexible and approach the target area by another route. This may require the patient to be in a position that the operator is not used to. For example, patients with pancreatic cancer may not be able to lie on their stomach but an anterior approach to coeliac plexus is a well-documented approach. Neurolytic intercostal nerve blocks may be performed with the patient in the lateral position.

Use of pillows and props may make the whole experience more tolerable for the patient. Use of assistance to get the patient into position is very useful. Log roll of patients will help to reduce pain during positioning. It may be necessary to give sedation and additional analgesia before undertaking the intervention, including positioning. Working with a team will facilitate and expedite this process.

Intervention support

Radiology technicians

Working with an experienced technician will make the procedure safer and a better experience for all parties. Clarify expectations with the technician, but do not compromise safety for speed.

A good radiographer will be able to position the C-arm quickly and correctly, identifying the target site efficiently. Always check the correct site and side before any injection is made.

If you are planning a CT-guided neurolytic coeliac plexus block and are not experienced in interpreting images, working with a radiologist is invaluable. The same is true when performing CT-guided trigeminal nerve block with alcohol.

Timeout

Before all interventional procedures, a timeout is mandatory. All parties in the suite must agree that the patient has been identified correctly, the procedure is correct, the site and side have been marked before sedation, and checked before injection. In addition, any other safety concerns need to be identified and documented. This would include: presence of dye allergy that has been addressed and identification of pacemaker and means to inactivate pacemaker if electrocautery is being used. We may be under pressure to get the procedure completed quickly, but these precautions will help to reduce any mishaps.

Assistance

Well-trained assistance during the procedure allows for smooth operations. Since each physician has personal preferences for various procedures, having premade procedure cards are helpful. One should identify the needles and various syringes needed as well as the medication to be injected. All syringes must be clearly marked to prevent any confusion. If a neurolytic agent is to be administered, it is vital that it be clearly marked and that the agent not be placed on the field before it is required. This will help to prevent any disasters.

Intervention procedure

Procedure

When performing any procedure on cancer patients, considerations need to include whether it is necessary to perform local anaesthetic block. Local anaesthetic block performed before a neurolytic block may be informative to see if the procedure is likely to be helpful, but will require the patient to have two separate procedures. A short spinal opioid trial before placement of an intrathecal catheter and pump must clearly identify benefits including better analgesia and reduction in side effects. Cancer patients with longer life expectancy may benefit from a longer trial as the main purpose of the trial in the latter category is to evaluate improved function and quality of life.

During the procedure

Be gentle. Use small-bore needles and inject medications slowly and incrementally. Be prepared to inject generous quantities of local anaesthesia. When neurolytic agents are injected, please ensure that adequate local anaesthetic has been administered before the injection to prevent pain with injection, done slowly and in small increments. Agents need to be clearly identified in the syringe and drawn up only before injection. If performing any spinal procedure like intrathecal administration of alcohol, please communicate with the patient, and ensure that no major nerves are being affected. If any injection is painful, stop and reassess. It may be necessary to reposition the needle, give more local anaesthetic, or even abandon the procedure. During these procedures, it may be necessary to provide sedation. Minimal sedation may be adequate. It is mandatory that monitoring be performed by a nurse trained in conscious sedation.

Postprocedure care

There is risk associated with these procedures and complications are bound to happen sooner or later. It is mandatory that all patients have follow-up appointments after any procedure. Some procedures need more intense follow-up than others. After a coeliac plexus block, patients' vitals need to be monitored, as hypotension is quite common. Adequate hydration is recommended.

Neurolysis of the ophthalmic division of the trigeminal nerve may cause loss of conjunctiva sensation resulting in corneal ulceration. It is important to give patients clear postoperative instructions, including eye care. They may need consultation with an ophthalmologist.

After a procedure patients may experience significant pain relief and this may necessitate rapid reduction of pain medications. Possibility of opioid withdrawal must be kept in mind.

Conclusion

Key learning points

- Interventional procedures are an integral part of the options available for treatment of certain cancer-related pain.
- A well-informed discussion must be undertaken so that expectations of patients, families, and caregivers are clearly defined.
- It is important to clearly document the plan for each patient. Documentation should include: the site, side of the body, and the intended procedure.
- Working with an experienced technician will make the procedure safer and a better experience for all parties.
- Before all interventional procedures, a timeout is mandatory. All parties in the suite must agree that the patient has been identified correctly, the procedure is correct, the site and side have been marked before sedation, and checked before injection.
- After a procedure patients may experience significant pain relief and this may necessitate rapid reduction of pain medications. Possibility of opioid withdrawal must be kept in mind.

Further reading

Cassell EJ (1982). The nature of suffering and the goals of medicine. *N Engl J Med*, **306**, 639–45.

Fishbain SM, Ballantyne JC, Rathmell JP (2010). *Bonica's Management of Pain*, 4th edn. Philadelphia, PA: Lippincott Williams and Wilkins.

Manchikanti L (2008). Evidence-based medicine, systematic reviews, and guidelines in interventional pain management, part 1: introduction and general considerations. *Pain Physician*, **11**(2), 161–86.

Van Norman GA, Jackson S, Rosenbaum SH, Palmer SK (2010). *Clinical Ethics in Anesthesiology: A Case-Based Textbook*. Cambridge: Cambridge University Press.

Sympathectomy for cancer pain

Dhanalakshmi Koyyalagunta and Arun Bhaskar

Introduction 148
Neurolysis 149
  Neurolytic agents 149
Coeliac plexus neurolysis 150
  Anatomy 150
  Neural connections 152
  Patient selection and indications 152
Techniques 153
  Evolution of the various techniques 153
  Classic technique 153
  Anterior approach 153
  Direct approach at surgery 153
  Transcrural coeliac plexus block 153
  Fluoroscopy-guided transcrural coeliac plexus block 154
  Retrocrural technique (splanchnic block) 154
  CT-guided coeliac plexus block 155
  Ultrasound-guided coeliac plexus block 157
Complications 158
Efficacy 159
  Key learning points 159
Superior hypogastric plexus neurolysis 160
  Anatomy 160
  Indications and patient selection 160
  Techniques 160
  Lateral approach 160
  Medial approach 160
  Transdiscal approach 161
  Anterior approach 162
  Complications 162
  Discussion 162
Ganglion impar block 163
  Anatomy 163
  Patient selection 163
  Classical technique 163
  Transcoccygeal approach 163
  Alternative approaches 165
  Complications 165
  Discussion 165
  Key learning points 165
Further reading 166

Introduction

Abdominal and pelvic pain in patients with malignancy can be debilitating and dramatically affects survival and quality of life. A meta-analysis showed a pooled pain prevalence of 59% in those with GI malignancy, 52% in those with urogenital malignancy, and 60% in those with gynaecological malignancy. Abdominal pain can be due to the tumour stretching, compressing, invading, or distending visceral structures, treatment-related tissue injury, radiation, or surgery. Patients typically describe the pain as deep, crampy, colicky, and vague in nature. The sympathetic and parasympathetic nervous system is involved in mediating visceral pain from the abdomen and pelvis. The autonomic nerves supplying the liver, pancreas, gall bladder, stomach, spleen, kidneys, adrenal glands, and part of the intestine (from the gastro-oesophageal junction to the splenic flexure of the colon) arise in the coeliac plexus.

The superior hypogastric plexus carries visceral nociceptive stimuli from the pelvic organs including the bladder, prostate, rectum, uterus, ovaries, and vagina.

The ganglion impar is an unpaired ganglion that marks the termination of the sympathetic chain; it carries visceral afferents from the distal rectum, anus, perineum, distal urethra, vagina, and vulva.

Treatment of abdominal and pelvic pain syndromes can be challenging. They are difficult to manage with oral analgesics adopting the WHO analgesic ladder alone. Patients with moderate to severe pain that is not controlled with oral analgesics or those who have medication-related side effects are ideal candidates for interventional therapies. Pain physicians and patients may need to seek interventional options early in the decision algorithm. Neurolytic sympathetic blocks should be considered as adjuvants to decrease the use of oral and/or parenteral analgesics and optimize pain control. However, it must be remembered that pain mechanisms in cancer are complex and change with progression of disease.

Neurolysis

Chemical neurolysis is widely used in the treatment of intractable cancer-related pain, the rationale being that these blocks will provide prolonged pain relief and decrease the need for oral pain medications. These blocks are associated with some morbidity, and it is prudent to understand the indications for each block to be able to select patients appropriately. There has been widespread acceptance of sympathetic neurolysis as, in the absence of rare, unexpected complications, this provides analgesia with no sensory or motor deficits. Diagnostic local anaesthetic blocks may be performed when indicated and possible, even before injecting neurolytic agent as one-stage procedure. Details of neurolysis and neurolytic agents are covered in Chapters 3 and 21.

Neurolytic agents

The agents currently used for chemical neurolysis are alcohol (50–100%), phenol (5–10%), and glycerol (50–100%). These agents disrupt transmission of pain signals by causing Wallerian degeneration distal to the lesion. They usually produce a block that lasts 3–6 months. Alcohol damages nerves by denaturing proteins, fatty substance extraction, and precipitation of lipoproteins and mucoproteins. Alcohol is hypobaric in comparison to CSF. It spreads rapidly from the injected site and larger volumes are required in comparison to phenol. It may be associated with neuritis. Alcohol is rapidly absorbed into the blood. Inadvertent intravascular injection may lead to thrombosis. Phenol has local anaesthetic properties at lower concentrations and it is a neurolytic agent at higher concentration. It is usually not painful on injection. Phenol diffuses into the axon and perineural blood vessels and denatures the proteins causing Wallerian degeneration with a relative sparing effect on the dorsal root ganglia. The intensity and duration of block with phenol is less than with alcohol and carries a lower risk of neuritis.

Coeliac plexus neurolysis

Anatomy

The coeliac plexus or the solar plexus is a diffuse network of nerve fibres and ganglia (1–5) that lies at the level of T12/L1 to the middle of L2 on the anterolateral surface of the aorta. It is the largest visceral plexus and comprises a dense network of interconnecting nerve fibres from the coeliac, superior mesenteric, and aorticorenal ganglia. It is a retroperitoneal structure and lies anterior to the crus of the diaphragm and inferior to the coeliac artery origin. Its anterior relationship includes the stomach and pancreas; posteriorly it is separated from the vertebral column by the diaphragmatic crura. The left ganglion is 0.9cm and the right ganglion is 0.6cm caudad to the coeliac artery. This relationship to the coeliac artery is relatively consistent and a reliable landmark for localizing the plexus (Figures 14.1–14.3).

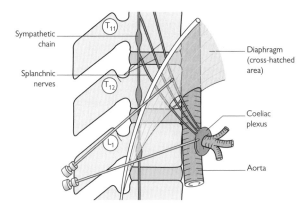

Figure 14.1 Diagram showing neural connections and various needle positions for coeliac plexus and splanchnic block. Image courtesy of Dr SG Tordoff FRCA FFPMRCA.

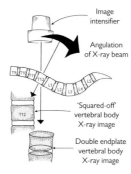

Figure 14.2 Diagram showing positioning of X-ray beam to square endplates of T12 for (retrocrural) splanchnic neurolysis (same projection can be used at L1 for coeliac plexus neurolysis). Image courtesy of Dr SG Tordoff FRCA FFPMRCA.

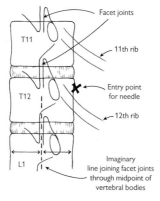

Figure 14.3 Diagram showing needle entry point for retrocrural (splanchnic) block at T12 (similar projection and needle entry point is used at L1 for coeliac plexus block). Image courtesy of Dr SG Tordoff FRCA FFPMRCA.

Neural connections

Sympathetic innervation to the abdominal viscera arises from preganglionic fibres from T5–T12 via the ventral roots. The roots unite to form the greater, lesser, and least splanchnic nerves that traverse the diaphragmatic crus to synapse with the coeliac plexus. The three splanchnic nerves are preganglionic and postganglionic fibres arising from the coeliac plexus supplying the abdominal viscera. Visceral afferents from the lower oesophagus, stomach, pancreas, liver, gall bladder, and parts of the intestine as far as the splenic flexure transmit pain through the splanchnic nerves and coeliac plexus. The coeliac plexus supplies parasympathetic, sympathetic, and visceral afferent fibres to these structures.

Patient selection and indications

Patients with cancer involving the viscera innervated by the coeliac plexus often present with upper abdominal pain radiating to the back. Those with intractable pain not relieved with opioids or who have medication-related side effects are ideal candidates for a coeliac plexus neurolysis (CPN). It is necessary to differentiate visceral from somatic pain from invasion of the musculoskeletal structures. Appropriate assessment and optimal patient selection will determine the outcome of the block.

There can be complications and undesirable side effects that should be discussed with the patient and their caregivers. Patients with uncorrectable coagulopathy and infection are not ideal candidates. CPN can cause unopposed parasympathetic activity and increase bowel motility and should be avoided when there is a concern for bowel obstruction. Review of scans for involvement of the coeliac plexus and extent of disease is necessary prior to the needle placement. There is decreased efficacy with nodal involvement and disease around the coeliac plexus.

Techniques

Blockade can be achieved by depositing local anaesthetic and/or neurolytic agent anterior to the aorta in the vicinity of the coeliac plexus or retro-crurally to block the splanchnic nerves. CPN decreases the need for oral analgesics, improves quality of life, and increases life expectancy in patients with unresectable pancreatic cancer.

Evolution of the various techniques

A percutaneous posterior approach to coeliac plexus blockade using bony landmarks was described by Max Kappis in 1914. Since then there has been significant evolution in the approaches and techniques, e.g. fluoroscopic-, CT-, ultrasound-, and endoscopic-guided techniques.

Classic technique

The 'classic technique' using bony landmarks was first described by Kappis and recounted by Labat (1924). This was done with the patient in the lateral decu-bitus position with the needle entry point below the 12th rib, 7cm from the spinous process. This required repositioning for injection on the opposite side. The needle was advanced towards the anterolateral margin of the vertebral body and 50–70mL of local anaesthetic was injected.

Anterior approach

An anterior percutaneous approach was described by Wendling in 1918 where the needle was introduced 1cm below the xiphoid process, 0.5cm to the left of the midline. The needle was advanced though the left lobe of the liver until it encountered the vertebral body usually at a depth of 6cm, where 50–80mL of local anaesthetic was injected. There was not much enthusiasm for this technique until a similar approach using CT guidance was described by Matamala in 1988. He injected neurolytic agent as well as proceeded with a biopsy in five patients.

Direct approach at surgery

Direct deposition of neurolytic agent during surgical laparotomy can be done and in the early 1920s coeliac plexus block at open laparotomy was described by Braun and Finsterer. Lillemoe et al. showed that patients with unresectable cancer had improved survival and pain relief with chemical sympathectomy at open laparotomy. Wiersema et al. first reported CPN with an endoscopic ultrasound-guided approach. It is an attractive option because it allows for a simultaneous tissue sampling.

Transcrural coeliac plexus block

Moore et al. used roentgenographic guidance for diagnostic blocks and performed CT-guided neurolysis. They concluded that needles should be placed bilaterally and at least 25mL of solution (either local anaesthetic or neurolytic agent) should be injected on each side. In 1982 Singler refined Moore's technique as he noted that with Moore's classic technique the nee-dle position was at times retrocrural and there was tracking of the neu-rolytic agent along the lumbar plexus. Ischia and colleagues described the transaortic approach to the coeliac plexus using a single needle with reliable deposition of neurolytic at the coeliac plexus. However, there is a potential risk for aortic dissection and tears and dislodgement of thrombus.

Fluoroscopy-guided transcrural coeliac plexus block

- This technique is performed by pain physicians in the operating (procedure) room setting.
- The patient is fasted and hydrated with 500–1000mL of intravenous fluid before the procedure. Routine monitoring is needed.
- The patient is prone on the procedure table.
- After sterile preparation and draping the vertebral bodies are identified using fluoroscopy.
- The C-arm is rotated 20–30° oblique until the tip of the transverse process of L1 overlies the anterolateral margin of L1 vertebrae.
- The skin and subcutaneous tissues are anaesthetized with local anaesthetic.
- A 22G 150mm needle is used; this can be modified depending on body habitus.
- A transaortic technique can be performed using a single needle from the left.
- The needle is advanced towards the anterolateral margin of the L1 vertebral body with frequent images in the anteroposterior (AP) and lateral views.
- Once the needle is positioned at the anterolateral margin of the L1 vertebral body, it is advanced 2–3 cm with fluoroscopy as well as continuous aspiration.
- Once blood is aspirated, the needle is advanced to pass anterior to the aorta until blood is no longer aspirated.
- The final needle position is confirmed by injecting contrast and seeing it spread anterior to the aorta.
- If there is not adequate spread across the midline to the right, a second needle should be placed on the opposite side.
- Diagnostic block with 10mL of 0.25% to 0.5% bupivacaine is performed and a total of 20mL of absolute alcohol or 10% phenol (neurolytic agent) is injected incrementally.

Retrocrural technique (splanchnic block)

- This is a modification of the transcrural technique and is performed at T11 or T12.
- The preprocedure preparation and patient positioning are similar.
- The fluoroscopy beam is rotated 20–30° oblique until the transverse process of T12 is flush with vertebral body.
- A 22G, 150mm needle is used.
- The needle is advanced to the anterolateral margin of the vertebral body with frequent imaging.
- Once the needle is at the anterolateral margin, it is advanced to the anterior border of the vertebral body in the lateral view.
- A similar needle is placed on the opposite side.
- After negative aspiration, contrast is injected to confirm spread over the anterior vertebral body and to ensure no posterior tracking.

- 5mL of 0.25% bupivacaine is injected for diagnostic purposes followed by 7–10mL of absolute alcohol (neurolytic agent) through each needle incrementally.
- Contrast can be mixed with neurolytic agent and local anaesthetic to improve comfort and safety.
- 2mL of local anaesthetic is injected to flush the neurolytic agent out of the needle, the stilette is replaced and the needle removed (Figures 14.4 and 14.5).

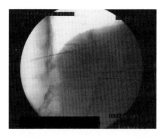

Figure 14.4 Showing retrocrural technique of splanchnic block.
Supplied by Dr Arun Bhaskar.

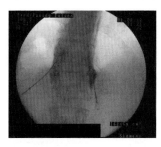

Figure 14.5 Showing retrocrural technique of splanchnic block.
Supplied by Dr Arun Bhaskar.

CT-guided coeliac plexus block

- Preprocedure preparation and monitoring are similar to the retrocrural and transcrural approaches.
- The most common CT-guided approach is posterior anterocrural performed with the patient in the prone position.
- A preliminary CT is performed to localize the coeliac artery, select the needle puncture site, and determine the angle and depth of needle entry.
- The optimum site of injection is between the superior mesenteric artery and the coeliac trunk.
- After sterile preparation and local anaesthesia, a 22G, 150mm needle is advanced into the subcutaneous tissue.

- With CT guidance the trajectory of the needle is changed toward the anterolateral surface of the aorta.
- The needle is advanced along the vertebral body, with care to avoid the rib, kidneys, and other vascular structures.
- Once the needle position is approximately 1–2cm anterior to the aorta, after negative aspiration, a small amount (0.5–1mL) of water-soluble non-ionic iodinated contrast is injected.
- A correct needle placement is indicated by contrast spread in the antecrural space. If the contrast spreads across the midline, the block can be performed with a single needle.
- Spread in at least three of the four quadrants has shown to provide long-lasting analgesic efficacy.
- The spread of the neurolytic agent may not be optimum with regional anatomical variations. 20mL of neurolytic agent can be injected in incremental doses (Figures 14.6 and 14.7).

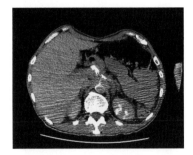

Figure 14.6 Showing landmarks for CT-guided coeliac plexus block.
Supplied by Dr Arun Bhaskar.

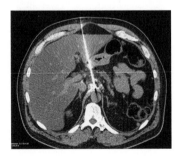

Figure 14.7 Showing needle in place for CT-guided coeliac plexus block.
Supplied by Dr Arun Bhaskar.

Ultrasound-guided coeliac plexus block

The ultrasound-guided, percutaneous, anterior approach is an option for patients who need a block at the bedside as a palliative measure. CT scans are reviewed for 'favourable anatomy' as defined by the feasibility of approaching the plexus with no nodal involvement. The patient is supine with routine monitoring and intravenous fluids. The ultrasound transducer is used to locate the origins of the coeliac trunk and the superior mesenteric artery. The transducer is then rotated to image the origin of the coeliac trunk and the common hepatic and splenic artery. A 22G, 150mm Chiba needle is advanced into the epigastrium on either side of the midline until the needle tip is between the aorta and the coeliac trunk. 10mL of local anaesthetic is injected after negative aspiration. This is followed by absolute alcohol. The sonograph is used to visualize the real-time spread of the neurolytic agent.

Complications

Complications related to CPN differ with the technique used. Ischia *et al.* compared the complications and efficacy of classic retrocrural, bilateral splanchnic, and transaortic techniques.

- Hypotension was more frequent with the retrocrural approach (50%) or splanchnic (52%) technique possibly from sympathetic neurolysis.
- The incidence of transient complications, e.g. haematuria, hiccoughing, interscapular back pain, reactive pleurisy, and dysaesthesia were similar in all three groups.
- There are reports of gastroparesis, gastric perforation, and retroperitoneal fibrosis.
- Although infrequent, paraplegia is one of the most devastating complications of neurolytic coeliac plexus block. The incidence appears to be <1:1000. The cause of paraplegia may be from the spread of neurolytic to the posterior surface of the aorta at the level of the spinal segmental arteries that can lead to spasm of the arteries that perfuse the spinal cord. The neurolytic agent can cause necrosis or occlusion of the artery of Adamkiewicz leading to paraplegia.
- The incidence of diarrhoea and hypotension was more frequent after an antecrural transaortic approach (65%). These are usually transient and to some extent hypotension can be prevented by adequate hydration. On occasions these problems can be prolonged requiring hospitalization and treatment with intravenous hydration. Orthostatic hypotension can last for up to 5 days. Treatment includes adequate hydration, bed rest with legs raised, elastic stockings, and avoidance of sudden changes in position. Diarrhoea can lead to severe dehydration in debilitated patients. Treatment includes aggressive hydration (oral or parenteral) and antidiarrhoeal agents.
- Renal injury and haematuria, intravascular injection, and pneumothorax are complications related to needle positioning. The use of CT or ultrasound guidance will allow visualization of the kidney and pleura and decrease the incidence of these complications. The transaortic approaches can lead to rupture or aortic dissection and haemorrhage. This technique should be avoided in patients with aortic atherosclerotic disease.
- Retroperitoneal haemorrhage is a rare complication and should be suspected when the patient complains of backache and hypotension after the block.
- Backache is frequently seen from needle trauma as well as alcohol-mediated irritation of retroperitoneal structures. Serial haematocrits should be performed for persistent backache to rule out retroperitoneal bleeding and radiological imaging should be used as indicated.

Alcohol is painful on injection and it is necessary to use local anaesthetic or provide sedation. Accidental intravascular injection of 30mL, 100% ethanol can lead to blood alcohol concentrations above the legal driving limit. Inadvertent intravascular injection of phenol can lead to manifestations similar to local anaesthetic toxicity including seizures and cardiovascular collapse. Tracking of neurolytic agent to the neuraxis or on to nerves can lead to neuritis.

Efficacy

A 2011 Cochrane review of CPN for pancreatic cancer pain concluded that 'although statistical evidence is minimal for the superiority of pain relief over analgesic therapy, the fact that CPB [coeliac plexus block] causes fewer adverse effects than opioids is important for patients'. Six studies with 358 subjects met the inclusion criteria (severe pain in patients with unresectable pancreatic cancer). Endoscopic-guided CPN provides detailed imaging of the blood vessels around the plexus and is theoretically superior to the fluoroscopic-guided posterior percutaneous approach, although there is a lack of comparative studies to prove this. Yan et al., in a systematic review (1966–2005), examined the efficacy and safety of CPN in randomized controlled trials. There were 302 patients in the five studies that met the inclusion criteria. CPN was associated with better pain control, decreased opioid requirement, and improvement in constipation. Survival rates were no different; it was difficult to assess change in quality of life due to different outcome scales used in each study.

Ischia et al. showed that patients with pancreatic cancer benefited from CPN early in the course of their disease when the pain was of 'coeliac type'; 70–80% of the patients had pain relief immediately after the block that was sustained in 60–75% cases until death. CPN alone was not adequate for complete pain relief, but showed substantial benefit by abolishing the visceral pain component. A study by De Cicco et al. assessed the analgesic benefit based on the injectate spread. Pain relief with a CT-guided anterior approach was dependent on neurolytic spread in four quadrants that was hampered by regional anatomic variations. 100% of patients had 'long-lasting' pain relief with spread in all four quadrants and this dropped to 48% with spread in three quadrants. None of the patients with injectate spread in one or two quadrants had any long-lasting pain relief.

Key learning points
- A variety of techniques are available for coeliac plexus block and hence the technique can be selected on patient choice, acceptability, local availability, and operator's choice.
- This block has high-quality evidence from randomized controlled trials to support reduction in opioid use and improved pain control in pancreatic cancer-related pain.
- Early offer of coeliac plexus block is more effective for pain control.
- Serious complications are very rare with use of image guidance and contrast injection before injection of neurolytic agent.
- The block can be repeated.

Superior hypogastric plexus neurolysis

Anatomy

The superior hypogastric plexus is retroperitoneal and lies on the anterior aspect of the L5 and S1 vertebral bodies below the aortic bifurcation. The sympathetic afferent and efferent fibres from the branches of the aortic plexus and splanchnic nerves form the plexus. The plexus is a continuation of coeliac and inferior mesenteric plexus. The superior hypogastric plexus converges and forms the hypogastric nerve distally. It innervates the pelvic visceral organs including the urinary bladder, prostate, uterus, vagina, and rectum. The hypogastric nerve follows the internal iliac vessels and joins the inferior hypogastric plexus. The plexus is predominantly left-sided so, if a single-needle technique is used, it should be targeted towards the left. The inferior hypogastric plexus is formed by the sympathetic fibres from the hypogastric nerves, postganglionic sympathetic fibres from sacral splanchnic nerves, and parasympathetic fibres from S2, S3, and S4; it lies close to the pelvic organs that it innervates.

Indications and patient selection

Superior hypogastric plexus block or neurolysis can provide good analgesia for patients with sympathetically mediated pain from pelvic visceral malignancy. Patients who have a pelvic mass inseparable from the urogenital organs arising from the urinary bladder, cervix/uterus, and rectum often benefit from the block. Effective blocks can significantly reduce the need for increasing doses of systemic opioids and improve quality of life by reducing the opioid-induced side effects. Contraindications include patient refusal, coagulopathy, and local/systemic infections. In patients with advanced disease the anatomy may be not be straightforward; risks and benefits should be carefully discussed with the patient.

Techniques

Plancarte et al. first reported the use of superior hypogastric plexus block. This was followed by description of laparoscopic, fluoroscopic, and CT-guided techniques for optimal needle placement. An anterior approach and transvaginal approach has been described. Most techniques including the transdiscal approach involve the patient being prone.

Lateral approach

The 'lateral' approach is the conventional technique with the patient in the prone position; a 20G, 150mm needle is introduced from a point lateral to the L4–L5 interspace medially and caudad parallel to the medial iliac border to just miss the sacral ala and L5 transverse process; the needle is then advanced to reach the anterior aspect of the L5 vertebral body; the final position is checked in the AP view to ensure that the needle is within 1cm of the bony outline of L5–S1.

Medial approach

- In the more popular medial approach (Figures 14.8 and 14.9), the patient is placed in the prone position with a pillow underneath the iliac crests and the fluoroscope C-arm is rotated 15° caudad to aim the X-ray beam 'into the pelvis' to identify the triangle formed by the transverse process of the L5 vertebra, the ala of the sacrum, and the posterior superior iliac spine.

- After adequate local anaesthesia to the skin, a 20G, 150mm needle is used to enter the inferior and lateral aspect of this space directing the needle caudad and medially under fluoroscopic guidance.
- When the needle passes the transverse process, the lateral view is used to confirm that the needle is passing above the L5 neural foramen and it is pushed in gently to reach the anterior border of the L5 vertebral body.
- In the AP view, the needle should be close to the bony outline of L5–S1.
- After negative aspiration the position is further confirmed with 3–5mL of water-soluble contrast medium, the spread of which should be limited to within the lateral bony margin above the sacral nerve roots and anterior to the psoas.
- Neurolysis may be carried out using 5mL of 6–10% aqueous phenol or 50–75% alcohol, monitoring the spread of the contrast.
- Often the blocks are carried out bilaterally and it is best to position both needles before injecting the contrast medium.

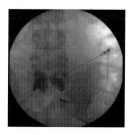

Figure 14.8 Needles in place for hypogastric plexus block, AP view.

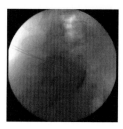

Figure 14.9 Needles in place for hypogastric plexus block, lateral view.

Transdiscal approach

- For the transdiscal approach the patient is placed prone with a pillow under the iliac crests.
- After aligning the endplates, the C-arm is rotated to visualize the L5–S1 intervertebral space and the disc.
- After local anaesthesia to the skin, a 22G, 100mm or 150mm needle is introduced under tunnel vision inferolateral to the ipsilateral facet joint line to enter the disc.

- It is best to confirm the angle of the alignment of the endplates of the L5 and S1 vertebral bodies on the lateral view so that the angle of the needle can be adjusted.
- Once the needle is in the disc, it is slowly advanced under lateral fluoroscopic view until the tip is anterior to the vertebral body.
- Loss of resistance to air or saline may be used to facilitate this, but final position should always be confirmed using 3–5mL water-soluble contrast under continuous fluoroscopy.
- Once this is confirmed, neurolytic block can be carried out using 5mL 6–10% aqueous phenol or 50–75% alcohol.
- The needle is withdrawn after a flush with 0.5mL normal saline.

Anterior approach

The anterior approach is not commonly used due to a high risk of hollow viscus perforation and infection. It may also be limited by the presence of a large pre-sacral mass. The patient is placed in 15° Trendelenburg in the supine position and L5 vertebral body is identified using ultrasound, fluoroscopy, or even by direct palpation in thin individuals. An 22G, 80mm spinal needle is introduced onto the anterior aspect of L5–S1 vertebral body, keeping it perpendicular to all planes. On negative aspiration, contrast is injected to ascertain the spread and about 10mL of neurolytic agent.

Complications

- The risk of inadvertent puncture of iliac vessels and intravascular injections are potential complications due to the close proximity of these vessels.
- The risk of haematoma following this or accidental injection of neurolytic into psoas can result in paraspinal muscle spasm and pain.
- The risk of major neurological sequelae is very rare, but neurolytic agent can track down and damage the L5 and sacral roots resulting in foot drop.
- Patients need to be warned about potential bowel and/or bladder dysfunction as well as potential loss of sexual function prior to the procedure.
- There is the risk of ureteral damage and intraperitoneal injection. The risk of infection is as with any interventional procedure, but discitis is relevant if the transdiscal approach is used. The risk is quite low at 1–4%, but most practitioners use prophylactic antibiotics.

Discussion

Even in early studies there was reduction in pain and no major complications after this procedure for pain due to malignancy of pelvic viscera. This was confirmed by Erdine *et al.* using the transdiscal technique; it was also noted that there was significant reduction in daily analgesic requirements. Plancarte and De Leon-Casasola in the largest study to date of 227 patients found that neurolytic superior hypogastric plexus block was efficacious (50% pain relief lasting at least 3 weeks and 40% reduction in use of opioid analgesics) in 51% of patients; however, when narrowing down to 159 patients who responded to diagnostic blocks, the success rate was 72% and with a mean reduction in concomitant analgesia of 43%. Studies and case series from several centres confirm that the risk of major complications is quite small.

Ganglion impar block

Anatomy

Ganglion impar, also known as the sacrococcygeal ganglion or ganglion of Walther, is the most caudal part of the sympathetic chain and is formed by fusion of the sympathetic ganglia from either side to form a single ganglion. It is often found anterior to the sacrococcygeal junction. Visceral afferents from vulva, perineum, and distal aspects of the urethra, vagina, and ano-rectum are relayed to the ganglion impar.

Patient selection

Blockade of the ganglion impar can be used to confirm whether pain in the perineum, rectum, or the vulvo-vagina is sympathetically mediated; if the diagnostic block is confirmatory, then neurolysis of the ganglion can be beneficial in patients with pelvic tumours of urogenital origin as well as ano-rectal cancers. Ganglion impar blocks provide good pain relief in patients with radiation proctitis.

Classical technique

- The original technique described by Plancarte et al. places the patient in the lateral decubitus position.
- After local anaesthetic infiltration of the skin overlying the ano-coccygeal ligament, found midway between the anal opening and the tip of the coccyx, a 22G spinal needle bent according to the coccygeal curvature is introduced in the midline and advanced to the sacrococcygeal junction (Figure 14.10).
- This can be facilitated by a finger in the rectum, which would then guide the needle; this reduces the risk of rectal perforation, but can compromise the aseptic technique and is uncomfortable for patients with rectal or pelvic pathology.

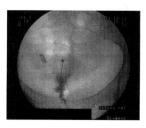

Figure 14.10 Needle in place with contrast for ganglion impar block, AP view.

Transcoccygeal approach

- The transcoccygeal approach (Figures 14.11 and 14.12) in the prone position involves introducing a 22G spinal needle in the midline at the sacrococcygeal junction through the coccygeal ligament.
- The needle is placed in its final position in the lateral view that is confirmed using 1–2mL contrast.

- This may be difficult in patients with severe arthritis or calcified ligaments.
- In this situation a paramedian approach can be used. A bent 22G spinal needle is inserted inferior and lateral to the sacral hiatus in the AP view and advanced in the lateral view until the needle tip is parallel to the sacrococcygeal ligament in the perirectal space.
- If bone is contacted prior to this, the needle can be gently re-directed.
- A lateral approach is also described where the needle is advanced below the transverse process of the coccyx to end in the midline just inferior to the sacrococcygeal junction.
- The advantage of this technique is that the patient may be prone or lateral and it is relatively easy in the presence of calcified ligaments.

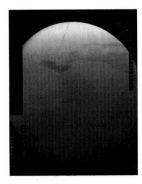

Figure 14.11 Needle in place with contrast for ganglion impar block, lateral view.

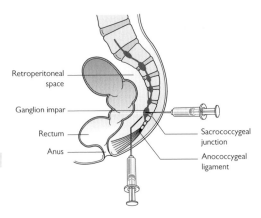

Retroperitoneal space

Ganglion impar

Rectum

Anus

Sacrococcygeal junction

Anococcygeal ligament

Figure 14.12 Spinal interventions in pain management. Image courtesy of Dr SG Tordoff FRCA FFPMRCA.

Alternative approaches

- A third approach for this block is with the patient in the lithotomy position using rectal finger to guide a 22G spinal needle to position, as the lithotomy position straightens the curvature of the coccyx.
- Ultrasound-guided techniques have been described. After confirming satisfactory needle position in the midline with any of the earlier described approaches, chemical neurolysis is carried out with 3–5mL of 6–10% aqueous phenol, monitoring the spread of contrast.
- RFA of the ganglion using thermal lesions has been described using single or double RF probes placed through the sacrococcygeal ligament and between Cx1 and Cx2 disc after appropriate sensory and motor testing.

Complications

- Ganglion impar block is relatively safe, but there is a risk of rectal puncture and infection, as well as injection of neurolytic into the rectal wall or cavity.
- Injection of neurolytic agent into the sacral nerve roots can cause neuritis and autonomic disturbances to the bowel and bladder function. The risk of major neurological sequelae is very rare.

Discussion

The location of the ganglion impar is varied and hence the success of the block depends on precise needle placement under fluoroscopy or CT guidance. Several studies have confirmed its safety and efficacy in managing perineal pain due to malignancy, but these are limited to case series and not randomized clinical trials.

Key learning points

- Superior hypogastric and ganglion impar block are of use in medically refractory pelvic and perineal pain.
- Complications are rare with use of fluoroscopy and contrast injection under continuous fluoroscopy.

Further reading

Agarwal-Kozlowski K, Lorke DE, Habermann CR, Am Esch JS, Beck H (2009). CT-guided blocks and neuroablation of the ganglion impar (Walther) in perineal pain: anatomy, technique, safety, and efficacy. *Clin J Pain*, 25(7), 570–6.

Arcidiacono PG, Calori G, Carrara S, McNicol ED, Testoni PA (2011). Celiac plexus block for pancreatic cancer pain in adults. *Cochrane Database Syst Rev*, 16(3), CD007519.

Burton AW, Hamid B (2007). Current challenges in cancer pain management: does the WHO ladder approach still have relevance? *Expert Rev Anticancer Ther*, 7, 1501–2.

Burton AW, Phan PC, Cousins MJ (2009). Treatment of cancer pain: role of neural blockade and neuromodulation. In Cousins MJ, Carr DB, Horlocker TT, Bridenbaugh PO (eds) *Cousins and Bridenbaugh's Neural Blockade in Clinical Anesthesia and Pain Medicine*, 4th edn, pp. 1111–54. Philadelphia, PA: Wolters Kluwer, Lippincott Williams & Wilkins.

De Cicco M, Matovic M, Bortolussi R, Coran F, Fantin D, Fabiani F, *et al.* (2001). Celiac plexus block: injectate spread and pain relief in patients with regional anatomic distortions. *Anesthesiology*, 94(4),561–5.

Erdine S, Yucel A, Celik M, Talu GK (2003). Transdiscal approach for hypogastric plexus block. *Reg Anesth Pain Med*, 28, 304–8.

Huang JJ (2003). Another modified approach to the ganglion of Walther block (ganglion of impar). *J Clin Anesth*, 15(4), 282–3.

Ischia S, Ischia A, Polati E, Finco G (1992). Three posterior percutaneous celiac plexus block techniques. A prospective, randomized study in 61 patients with pancreatic cancer pain. *Anesthesiology*, 76, 534–40.

Koyyalagunta D, Burton AW (2010). The role of chemical neurolysis in cancer pain. *Curr Pain Headache Rep*, 14, 261–7.

Lillemoe KD, Cameron JL, Kaufman HS, Yeo CJ, Pitt HA, Sauter PK (1993). Chemical splanchnicectomy in patients with unresectable pancreatic cancer. A prospective randomized trial. *Ann Surg*, 217, 447–55.

Moore DC, Bush WH, Burnett LL (1981). Celiac plexus block: a roentgenographic, anatomic study of technique and spread of solution in patients and corpses. *Anesth Analg*, 60, 369–79.

Plancarte R, De Leon-Casasola O (2005). Superior hypogsatric plexus block and ganglion impar (Walther). *Tech Reg Anesth Pain*, 9, 86–90.

van den Beuken-van Everdingen MH, de Rijke JM, Kessels AG, Schouten HC, van Kleef M, Patijn J (2007). Prevalence of pain in patients with cancer: a systematic review of the past 40 years. *Ann Oncol*, 18, 1437–49.

Wong GY, Schroeder DR, Carns PE, Wilson JL, Martin DP, Kinney MO, *et al.* (2004). Effect of neurolytic celiac plexus block on pain relief, quality of life, and survival in patients with unresectable pancreatic cancer: a randomized controlled trial. *JAMA*, 291, 1092–99.

Yan BM, Myers RP (2007). Neurolytic celiac plexus block for pain control in unresectable pancreatic cancer. *Am J Gastroenterol*, 102, 430–8.

Vertebroplasty and kyphoplasty in spinal metastasis pain

Kumar S. V. Das and Shubhabrata Biswas

Introduction *168*
Advantages *169*
  Pathophysiology and proposed mechanism of pain relief *169*
  Patient selection and imaging *169*
  Magnetic resonance imaging *169*
  Computed tomography scan *170*
  Isotope bone scan *171*
Contraindications *172*
  Absolute *172*
  Relative *172*
Procedure *173*
  Technique *173*
Complications *175*
  Cement leakage and cord compression *175*
  Pulmonary embolism and paradoxical cerebral embolism *175*
  Infection *175*
  Fracture *175*
  Collapse of adjacent vertebral body *175*
  Bleeding *176*
  Allergic reaction to cement *176*
Kyphoplasty *177*
Vertebroplasty with tumour ablative therapy *178*
Conclusion *179*
  Key learning points *179*
Further reading *180*

Introduction

Percutaneous vertebroplasty (PV) is a minimally invasive vertebral augmentation procedure in which bone cement, usually polymethylmethacrylate (PMMA), is injected under radiological guidance. The aim is to provide pain relief and stabilization to a vertebra which is partially collapsed or at the risk of collapse. Percutaneous acrylic cement injection was first reported by Galibert in 1987 for the treatment of painful aggressive haemangiomas. Since then over the years there has been marked development in delivery devices and PMMA types and modification of the technique. PV has now evolved as the treatment of choice for painful osteoporotic fractures refractory to medical management. Painful vertebral metastatic fractures, including myeloma, are the second most common indication for PV.

The findings of two randomized controlled trials demonstrated that for vertebroplasty in osteoporosis, the benefit of a placebo (local anaesthetic with sham procedure) is as good as vertebroplasty in pain reduction, at least in the short term. However, with regard to PV in malignancy there is a lack of good quality, robust data. A more recent large prospective study by Chew et al., showed reduction in pain and improvement in disability due to intractable pain from myeloma and spinal metastases.

NICE supports the use of PV as a procedure for pain relief in vertebral tumours. However, PV in advanced spinal disease is technically challenging and therefore has not been widely adopted.

Advantages

Several advantages of PV over the conventional modalities of pain relief viz. pharmacotherapy, radiotherapy, and open surgical stabilization have been described.

Medical management of pain due to vertebral metastasis may take a longer time to take effect and certain fractures may be refractory to medical treatment. Radiotherapy may be associated with harmful effects on the adjacent neural structures and the analgesic effect may not be immediate. Radiotherapy also does not enhance vertebral strength or stabilization. An open surgical stabilization procedure may not be a realistic option in a patient with spinal metastasis due to overall high surgical risk of intervention and general anaesthesia. Under these circumstances PV provides the following advantages:

- Minimally invasive
- Limited hospital stay
- General anaesthesia not necessary
- Early pain relief
- Antineoplastic agents used as radiosensitizers prior to radiotherapy are not required
- Can be used along with conventional antitumour therapy and radiotherapy
- Can be combined with biopsy and tumour ablative procedures.

Pathophysiology and proposed mechanism of pain relief

Mechanism of pain relief may be multifactorial. Vertebral augmentation techniques stabilize fractures and reduce the movement by microfractures and thereby reduce pain. However, the analgesic affect is not significantly affected by the volume of PMMA used. It is therefore suggested that the pain relief is also due to destruction of sensitive nerve endings by the heat generated by PMMA polymerization. Experimental data also suggest that cement itself is cytotoxic to nerve tissue and causes a neurolytic effect.

Patient selection and imaging

The importance of a multidisciplinary approach in selecting patients for spinal augmentation cannot be overemphasized. It is necessary that decision-making is based on input from the referring clinician, radiologist, spinal surgeon, and the pain management team. Detailed history and clinical examination are important to ascertain the cause of pain and exclude the other causes of pain. Radicular pain will need nerve root block and is not an indication for vertebroplasty.

The aims of imaging are to diagnose the cause of pain, the age of fracture, identify the level(s), exclude other causes of pain, and delineate the fracture anatomy. It is particularly important to exclude involvement of the posterior vertebral body wall. The imaging modalities employed are as follows.

Magnetic resonance imaging

Axial and sagittal T1-weighted (Figure 15.1), T2-weighted (Figure 15.2), and STIR (short tau inversion recovery) images are obtained to confirm a pathological fracture secondary to malignancy. The signal characteristics also provide information about the age of the fracture. Other causes including infection should be excluded. Extent of the fracture and involvement of the nerve roots can also be identified.

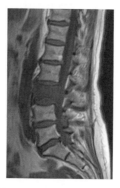

Figure 15.1 Patient with lung cancer presenting with back pain. Sagittal T1-weighted image.

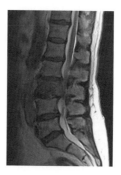

Figure 15.2 Patient with lung cancer presenting with back pain. T2-weighted image showing metastasis to the L3 vertebral body.

Computed tomography scan

Localized CT scan can be performed to delineate the fracture anatomy. This is particularly helpful in determining the integrity of the posterior vertebral body wall (Figure 15.3). The degree of compression can more accurately be measured by CT. CT also demonstrates extension of fracture into the posterior elements and resultant bony narrowing of the nerve root foramina.

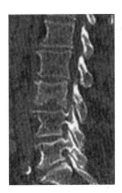

Figure 15.3 Computed tomography with sagittal reformat. Lucent areas seen within L3 vertebral body with intact posterior margin.

Isotope bone scan

The main benefit of isotope bone scan is to determine the age of the fracture. A relatively recent fracture will demonstrate more photopaenia and better outcome with augmentation techniques.

Contraindications

Several contraindications—absolute and relative—have been described.

Absolute

- Asymptomatic vertebral body involvement
- Pain improvement on conservative therapy
- Spondylodiscitis or any active systemic infection
- Uncontrolled coagulopathy
- Allergy to bone cement.

Relative

- Radicular pain.
- Tumour extension into the vertebral canal or cord compression. In epidural extension of tumour with neurological compromise PV may be combined with radiation treatment. Potentially complex surgical fixation procedures requiring an anterior approach can be simplified by combining PV with laminectomy.
- Posterior column disruption. Although associated with an increased risk of cement leak, PV has been frequently performed with success in patients with posterior column involvement.
- Vertebral body collapse of >70%, as needle insertion and placement may be difficult.
- Significant spinal canal stenosis due to retropulsed tumour or bone fragment.
- Patients with more than five metastases or diffuse metastases without clear pain level.
- Lack of surgical backup—in cases of symptomatic cement leakage in spinal canal.

Procedure

The Society of Interventional Radiology and the Cardiovascular and Interventional Radiological Society of Europe have put forward guidelines for quality assurance and improvement.

Informed consent is obtained following discussion with the patient and family (if agreed by the patient) with regard to the procedure, benefits, and complications. Anaphylaxis and death from PMMA as a rare complication also need to be discussed. Patients should also be consulted about the possibility of failure of pain relief and the need for open surgical stabilization.

Full blood count and coagulation screen should be performed prior to the procedure. Inflammatory markers including C-reactive protein (CRP) are checked to exclude underlying infection.

Preprocedural anaesthetic assessment should also be arranged.

Technique

PV can be performed under local anaesthesia in combination with conscious sedation. General anaesthesia is used in patients who are less likely to cooperate or remain agitated. Pulse, oxygen saturation, and blood pressure are monitored throughout the procedure.

The procedure is performed in sterile and strictly aseptic conditions. Intraoperative antibiotic cover is recommended in immunocompromised patients, but whether other patients should have this cover is often an individual decision. We routinely give broad-spectrum antibiotics as prophylaxis.

The procedure is performed under bi-plane fluoroscopic guidance. Dual guidance using CT and fluoroscopy can be employed in difficult cases. The operator should therefore have a detailed knowledge and training in use of the imaging techniques. The operator should also be able to interpret the preoperative images obtained and have full knowledge of the anatomy of the affected vertebra(e) so as to plan the procedure appropriately.

A transpedicular route is employed for lumbar spine. In the thoracic spine a transpedicular or a costovertebral route is adopted. An anterolateral approach is used for cervical spine. The patient is placed prone for thoracic and lumbar spinal procedures and supine for cervical spine. The approach can be mono- or bi-pedicular.

Various PV kits are commercially available which come with the needles and cement delivery devices besides the components of the cement. An 11–13G bone biopsy needle is typically used. Using AP (Figure 15.4) and lateral fluoroscopy (Figure 15.5), the needle tip is placed in the anterior part of the vertebral body. Venography by injecting 1–3mL of iodinated contrast may be performed to identify potential routes of cement extravasation. This is, however, not generally performed as results are variable and often do not mimic the behaviour of PMMA.

The cement is prepared once the needle is in position. The older generation cements used an opacifying agent like barium sulphate. However, radio-opacity is an important feature of new-generation cements. Once the cement assumes a toothpaste-like consistency, it is ready to be injected.

Injection is performed under continuous lateral and intermittent AP fluoroscopy to detect cement leak. In case of cement leak waiting for 30–60 seconds will harden the cement and often seal the leak. The position or direction of the needle tip is altered if the leak continues. Injection is continued till at least two-thirds of the vertebral body is filled homogenously between the endplates.

The patient is mobilized after 2 hours of bed rest. The vital parameters and the neurological signs are evaluated closely. In case of any deterioration of neurological status, assessment of cement leak and cord or nerve root compression is made with a CT scan.

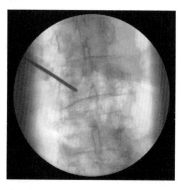

Figure 15.4 Vertebroplasty using unilateral transpedicular approach.

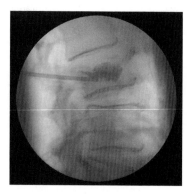

Figure 15.5 PMMA injection into the lumbar vertebral body.

Complications

Complications from PV for malignant fractures have been quoted to be higher than in PV for osteoporotic fractures (<10% vs <1%).

Cement leakage and cord compression

Asymptomatic cement leakage is not uncommon. Cement leakage has been reported in up to 41% of PV procedures but is rarely symptomatic.

However, cement leakage during PV in metastatic spine has been reported to be higher than in osteoporotic spine. The injection of bone cement into a vertebral body with metastatic tumour is typically more difficult than injection into an osteoporotic vertebra and the increased risk of leak may be related both to the increased pressure generated and associated bone destruction.

Cement leakage into the epidural space can occur, causing cord compression and paraplegia. Cement leakage through the neural foramina can result in radiculopathy due to nerve root compression.

Transient neurological deficit occurs in 5% of patients with malignant aetiology (compared to 1% in osteoporotic patients). The incidence of permanent neurological deficit (>30 days) in neoplastic aetiology is 2%.

Cord compression requires surgical decompression. In case of leakage into the nerve root foramina, cooling the nerve root by injecting normal saline into the foramina by a spinal needle may reduce the thermal effect of cement on the nerve root.

Cement leak into the disc space and paravertebral tissues is usually without any clinical consequence. However, large leak into the discs with a background of osteoporosis may lead to collapse of adjacent vertebral bodies.

Pulmonary embolism and paradoxical cerebral embolism

Cement leakage into paravertebral venous plexus can lead to pulmonary emboli, most of which are minimally symptomatic. Lethal pulmonary emboli and paradoxical cerebral embolism have also been reported. Invasion of cement in the inferior vena cava, lungs, heart, and even kidneys have been described.

Infection

Incidence is <1%. Several cases of osteomyelitis have been reported. These may require surgical intervention in the form of debridement and corpectomy.

Fracture

Incidence of fracture of pedicle or posterior elements has been reported in less than 1% of cases.

Collapse of adjacent vertebral body

New fractures involving mainly the immediate adjacent levels have been reported, varying between 7% and 20%, with a relative risk of 4.62 for fractures adjacent to the treated level versus fractures at the non-adjacent level. Altered biomechanics following PV has been attributed as the possible cause of the adjacent level fracture. However, a prospective observational study by Al-Ali *et al.* in 357 successive patients demonstrated the incidence of an adjacent vertebral compression fracture at 1 year or less after PV was comparable with that expected for untreated osteoporotic fractures.

Bleeding

Bleeding at the puncture site is usually minor and reduced by compression. Risk of bleeding is greater in vascular lesions (metastases from renal cell carcinoma and thyroid carcinoma) or if multiple levels are targeted.

Allergic reaction to cement

Anaphylactic death from PMMA has been reported.

Kyphoplasty

Kyphoplasty is a vertebral augmentation technique in which a height restoration device in the form of an inflatable balloon ('balloon tamp') is inserted percutaneously into the vertebral body and inflated with liquid. The Cancer Fracture and Evaluation (CAFÉ) study demonstrated the efficacy of kyphoplasty in pain reduction and improvement of function when compared with non-surgical management. Besides pain relief and enhancing the mechanical strength of the vertebral body, the idea of kyphoplasty is to correct kyphosis and restore vertebral height. The inflation of the balloon creates a cavity within the vertebral body. The balloon is deflated and the cavity is then filled with PMMA.

Kyphoplasty can be performed under conscious sedation or general anaesthesia. Using bi-planar fluoroscopy or under CT guidance the balloon is placed in the appropriate position. The cannula is inserted into the posterior aspect of the vertebral body by either a uni- or bilateral approach.

Typically there is little discernible restoration of height in most cases. However, there is evidence for lower incidence of cement leakage which has been reported as ranging from 0–33%. It has been suggested that controlled cement injection into the cavity created by balloon inflation as well as encasement of the cavity by the shell of impacted cancellous bone reduces the possibility of cement leak.

Kyphoplasty can be up to 10× more expensive than vertebroplasty. Although the CAFÉ trial demonstrated the benefit of kyphoplasty over conservative management, the trial did not answer important questions regarding patients with cancer. Careful consideration needs to be made regarding the effect of balloon compression in metastatic vertebral fractures which have weak bones and contain expressible soft tissue. It has also been noted previously that kyphoplasty was associated with the higher number of surgical decompressions for spinal compression.

With minimal to no height restoration in majority of cases, the relatively lower rate of cement leakage appears to be the only factor favouring the use of kyphoplasty over vertebroplasty.

Vertebroplasty with tumour ablative therapy

Radiofrequency ablation (RFA) can be combined with PV. Under CT guidance the RF electrode is inserted into the vertebra and activated. The heat generated causes cell destruction. Vertebral augmentation is performed at the same sitting. An intact posterior cortex is important to insulate the spinal cord from the heat generated by RFA.

Plasma-based RF ionization similarly can be employed in tandem with PV. The procedure employs RF energy in a conductive medium to produce a focused plasma field which has sufficient energy to break molecular bonds and cause dissolution of soft tissues at a relatively lower temperature (40–70°C). The procedure thereby creates a cavity by dissolution of the tumour cells rather than displacement reducing the risk of cement leakage and involving minimal deposition of heat in the spine. The procedure has been proposed as being safer and more appropriate for patients with posterior cortical defect.

Conclusion

Key learning points

- A recent large prospective study by Chew *et al.* showed reduction in pain and improvement in disability due to intractable pain from myeloma and spinal metastases.
- The Society of Interventional Radiology and the Cardiovascular and Interventional Radiological Society of Europe have prepared guidelines for quality assurance and improvement.
- The importance of a multidisciplinary approach in selecting patients for spinal augmentation cannot be overemphasized.
- NICE supports the use of PV as a procedure for pain relief in vertebral tumours.

Further reading

Arghayev K, Papanastassiou ID, Vrionis F (2011). Role of vertebral augmentation procedures in the management of vertebral compression fractures in cancer patients. *Curr Opin Support Palliat Care*, 5, 222–6.

Buchbinder R, Osborne RH, Ebeling PR, Wark JD, Mitchell P, Wriedt C, et al. (2009). A randomized trial of vertebroplasty for painful osteoporotic vertebral fractures. *N Eng J Med*, 361, 557–68.

Chew C, Ritchie M, O'Dwyer PJ, Edwards R (2011). A prospective study of percutaneous vertebroplasty in patients with myeloma and spinal metastases. *Clin Radiol*, 66, 1193–6.

Galibert P, Deramond H, Rosat P, Le Gars D (1987). Preliminary note on the treatment of vertebral angioma by percutaneous acrylic vertebroplasty. *Neurochirurgie*, 33(2), 166–8.

Gangi A, Buy X (2010). Percutaneous bone tumour management. *Semin Intervent Radiol*, 27, 124–36.

McGraw JK, Cardella J, Barr JD, Mathis JM, Sanchez O, Schwartzberg MS, et al. (2003). Society of Interventional Radiology quality improvement guidelines for percutaneous vertebroplasty. *J Vasc Interv Radiol*, 14, 827–31.

Tancioni F, Lorenzetti MA, Navarria P, Pessina F, Draghi R, Pedrazzoli P, et al. (2011). Percutaneous vertebral augmentation in metastatic disease: state of the art. *J Support Oncol*, 9, 4–10.

Cervical cordotomy for cancer pain

Manohar Sharma

Introduction *182*
Historical perspective *183*
Anatomical considerations *184*
Indications for percutaneous cervical cordotomy *187*
Contraindications *188*
Technique *189*
  Preparation *189*
  Equipment *189*
  Patient position *189*
  Imaging *190*
  Needle insertion *190*
  Myelogram *190*
  Inserting cordotomy probe into spinal cord *191*
  Radiofrequency lesion technique *191*
  Clinical pearls *191*
  Postcervical cordotomy aftercare *192*
  Efficacy of cervical cordotomy *192*
  Complications of cervical cordotomy *192*
Bilateral cordotomy *193*
  Future developments *193*
Conclusion *194*
  Key learning points *194*
Further reading *195*

Introduction

There is a growing interest in percutaneous cervical cordotomy (PCC) as an effective pain relief procedure in the UK because of an expected increase in mesothelioma cases. Various publications and manuals have recommended access to cordotomy services for selective indications with difficult to control cancer pain syndromes. Cordotomy is very effective as a palliative pain control procedure for unilateral, medically refractory cancer pain below the 4th cervical dermatome. Essentially, cervical cordotomy means RFA of spinothalamic tracts on the side contralateral to medically refractory cancer pain.

Historical perspective

PCC was introduced by Mullan and Rosomoff in the mid 1960s; this was an advance over open surgical cordotomy that was first described by Spiller and Martin in 1912. There was considerable morbidity and mortality attached to open cordotomy. In the 1960s, RF techniques were introduced to generate quick, uniform, and reliable heat lesions to the Gasserian ganglion. Initially PCC was used for a variety of indications including unilateral cancer pain, post-herpetic neuralgia, phantom limb pain, and post-stroke pain. However, the results were much better in unilateral, medically refractory cancer pain. Improvement in pharmacological treatments and the introduction of the WHO ladder for cancer pain in 1986 had decreased interest in cervical cordotomy. However, with improved understanding of the limitations of opioids in controlling many cancer pain syndromes and other side effects, cordotomy has now regained its place in a small number of carefully selected patients with complex unilateral cancer pain.

Anatomical considerations

PCC is carried out between the 1st and 2nd cervical foramina. This is the widest space and allows easy access to the intrathecal space and needle trajectory adjustments (Figures 16.1 and 16.2). It is carried out on the side opposite to the pain as pain fibres (spinothalamic tract) cross to the other side after entering the dorsal horn. Temperature sensation is also transmitted by these nerve fibres transmitting nociceptive pain. For this reason, it is very common for patients to have difficulty in perception of temperature on the affected half of the body following successful cordotomy. A lesion is carried out after localization of the spinothalamic tracts in the anterolateral quadrant of the spinal cord (Figures 16.3 and 16.4). On fluoroscopic images, the dentate ligament is seen to divide the spinal cord into anterior and posterior halves; this is easily visualized on myelogram through the 1st and 2nd cervical foramina (Figure 16.5). Sacral pain fibres are located superficially and adjacent to the dentate ligament; cervical fibres are deeper and more anterior (Figure 16.3). This anatomy is relevant when localizing a cordotomy RF probe in the anterolateral quadrant of spinal cord. The corticospinal tract is located posterior to the dentate ligament and if the cordotomy probe is close to it, motor stimulation at low thresholds will result in arm or leg movement on the ipsilateral side.

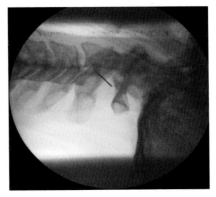

Figure 16.1 Initial needle insertion target point.

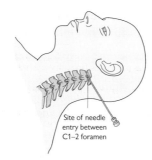

Figure 16.2 Diagram showing needle entry between 1st and 2nd cervical foramen. Image courtesy of Dr SG Tordoff FRCA FFPMRCA.

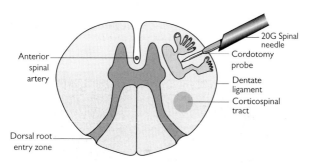

Figure 16.3 Cordotomy probe introduced through spinal needle into anterolateral quadrant of spinal cord. Image courtesy of Dr SG Tordoff FRCA FFPMRCA.

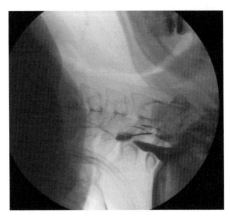

Figure 16.4 Cordotomy probe introduced through spinal needle into anterolateral quadrant of spinal cord.

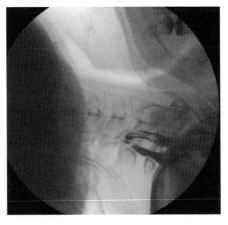

Figure 16.5 Needle just anterior to dentate ligament.

Indications for percutaneous cervical cordotomy

- Unilateral pain below the 4th cervical dermatome (below shoulder)
- Pain predominantly nociceptive (movement-related or incident pain)
- Satisfactory ventilatory reserve
- Expected survival >3 months and <1 year
- Medically refractory unilateral cancer pain (e.g. mesothelioma)
- Pain caused by cancer or metastases (confirmed tissue diagnosis)
- Very rarely considered for severe benign pain in a terminally ill patient (who is unsuitable for curative therapy).

Contraindications

Contraindications are very few, e.g. local infection, bleeding/clotting abnormalities, the patient's unacceptability of procedure, inability of the patient to cooperate, inability to lie supine for approximately 45 minutes, and poor ventilatory reserve.

Technique

Preparation

- Consent includes discussion of likely success rate and potential complications.
- All patients must be warned about the risks of failure of analgesia, motor weakness, sensory loss especially inability to discriminate temperature sensation in the area affected by cordotomy, bowel/bladder impairment, headache, neck pain, and feeling unwell for 24–48 hours after cordotomy.
- Prepare the patient as for general anaesthesia. Sedation is very often required. Intravenous access, oxygen administration by nasal speculae and routine monitoring is essential.
- Strict asepsis is essential. It is usual to administer one dose of prophylactic antibiotic according to local guidance.
- Another experienced team member must be dedicated to monitoring patient comfort and allay their anxiety related to procedure.

Equipment

X-ray machine, RF lesion generator, 20G 100mm spinal needle, cordotomy RF probe with 2mm active tip (Figure 16.6), oil-based or water-soluble radio-opaque contrast, local anaesthetic, and simple equipment for sensory examination after the heat lesion, e.g. ice cubes and neuro-tips.

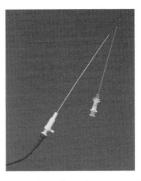

Figure 16.6 Spinal needle and disposable cordotomy probe. Reproduced courtesy of Minta® Medical Ltd and PAJUNK®.

Patient position

Position the patient supine on a radiolucent table with the head held in special head rest, the height of which can be adjusted (Figure 16.7). Head is held in position by straps so as to prevent extremes of neck movements.

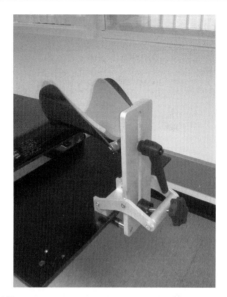

Figure 16.7 Cordotomy head rest. Reproduced courtesy of Wolverson X-Ray Limited, <http://www.wolverson.uk.com>.

Imaging

The C-arm should be positioned to obtain a lateral view of the cervical spine (Figure 16.1). Minor adjustments may be needed to clearly define the margins of the 1st and 2nd cervical foramina. The AP view should be checked during the procedure to minimize chances of the spinal needle crossing the midline.

Needle insertion

To find the target point the operator should imagine the boundaries of 1st and 2nd cervical foramina as the roof and walls of a hut. Needle entry point is on lamina of 2nd cervical vertebra where roof seems to join the walls of imaginary picture (Figure 16.1). Under local anaesthesia a 20G spinal needle is inserted between the 1st and the 2nd cervical vertebrae.

Myelogram

After free flow of CSF, a myelogram is obtained using a lipid-based radio-opaque or water-soluble contrast, e.g. 1–2mL of a 3mL mixture of lipoidal mixed with 8mL normal saline or CSF. Satisfactory myelogram shows the needle to be correctly positioned by visualizing dentate ligament (Figure 16.5). If the needle is posterior to dentate ligament, then the myelogram will not show the dentate ligament. In this situation the spinal needle has to be redirected anteriorly, so that its tip lies just anterior to dentate ligament. It is helpful at times to use needle supportive devices (Figure 16.8),

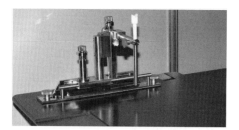

Figure 16.8 Cordotomy needle holder. Reproduced courtesy of Wolverson X-Ray Limited, <http://www.wolverson.uk.com>.

which can also be used to redirect needle to adjust its trajectory so as to enter anterolateral quadrant of spinal cord.

Inserting cordotomy probe into spinal cord

Once the correct image is obtained with the spinal needle just anterior to dentate ligament (Figure 16.5), the cordotomy probe is passed just anterior to the dentate ligament through the spinal needle into the anterolateral quadrant of spinal cord (Figure 16.4). The correct position of the electrode in the spinal cord is confirmed by sensory stimulation at 0.1V or less. Patients usually report severe burning or icy cold sensation in the contralateral side of body; this is usually below the shoulder area. On motor stimulation there should be no motor twitch on the ipsilateral side of the body, except in neck muscles at about 0.5V. If the probe tip is close to corticospinal tracts, then motor stimulation is ipsilateral. In some cases localizing the spinothalamic tract can be very difficult and painful or distressing to the patient. This is helped by sedation at this stage.

Radiofrequency lesion technique

Once satisfactory cordotomy probe position is confirmed, a gradual RF lesion is created in incremental steps, starting at 75°C and going up to 85°C. Each lesion is for 30 seconds. After each RF lesion, sensory and motor power testing is repeated to ensure demonstration of reduction in pin prick sensation (impairment of temperature discrimination) and no motor weakness. Small doses of opioid can be used to make RF lesioning less distressing. Patients usually report immediate and complete relief of pain. For beginners, it may be beneficial to have experienced colleagues in theatre including an experienced radiographer.

Clinical pearls

- Try to direct the spinal needle to the dural sac using an end-on or gun barrel approach. This maximizes chances of localizing the spinothalamic pathway.
- Once the spinal needle is intrathecal, make sure there is free flow of CSF. If not, there is a possibility of the spinal needle being in the substance of spinal cord or touching the surface of spinal cord.

- It may be worthwhile checking AP images through an open mouth view to see depth of needle/probe. There is no need to cross the midline (midline of odontoid peg).
- If, on first spinal needle insertion and myelogram, the spinal needle tip is too anterior (making cordotomy probe insertion in anterolateral quadrant of spinal cord difficult), then, it may be worth introducing another spinal needle in a position just anterior to the dentate ligament.
- It is beneficial to reduce opioid dose by half on the day of the procedure, particularly if the patient is taking very high doses; this helps to minimize opioid toxicity in the postprocedure period.
- One needs a very cooperative patient, patient operator, and experienced team for this procedure.

Postcervical cordotomy aftercare

The patient needs the usual postoperative care and can usually be discharged after 2 days. If there are concerns regarding infection, then oral or intravenous antibiotics are useful. It is important to have a patient care pathway that is helpful to nursing staff on the ward or hospice. It is vital to avoid any falls especially when patients are mobilized for the first time after cordotomy. The services of physiotherapist and occupational therapist can be of immense value, especially during the recovery phase.

Efficacy of cervical cordotomy

If patients are carefully selected, 75–80% find this procedure very effective for pain relief. It is usual to have a reduction in opioids and other analgesics by half. There is great improvement in quality of life in many patients. However, progression of the underlying cancer may still compromise quality of life. Similar results have been shown by author's prospective audit over 3 years.

Complications of cervical cordotomy

- It is very common to have headache and neck pain for a few days afterwards. Serious complications are rare. Ventilatory failure can occur, especially if the lesioning is for mesothelioma.
- Mirror pain is reported in about 10–15% of patients; it usually settles after a week or so; it is less severe than the original pain.
- Bowel and bladder weakness is more common after bilateral cordotomy and its incidence is around 5% for unilateral cervical cordotomy.
- Numbness, dysaesthetic sensation, and motor weakness are encountered in around 5–10% of patients; they usually cope very well.
- Very rarely death or serious catastrophic events can occur.
- As patients cannot discriminate between hot and cold sensation (e.g. a hot cup of tea held in the hand on the side affected by cordotomy will not feel hot). Burns have been described, if due care is not taken.

Bilateral cordotomy

Bilateral PCC has been described in literature and some practitioners still offer this in Europe as a staged procedure. The author prefers not to offer bilateral PCC because of perceived risks of Ondine's curse. If the patient develops severe pain on the side opposite to initial pain and if the pain is below T6 dermatome, then they are offered open surgical cordotomy at T1–T3 level. This is well tolerated as it is carried out under general anaesthesia, but there is a very high risk of bowel and bladder control impairment. This may be acceptable in a patient who is terminally ill and has very severe uncontrollable pain. Open bilateral surgical cordotomy has been described recently with good outcome for pain relief. Rarely, open surgical cordotomy can be offered to a patient who may not be able to tolerate PCC and if the pain is below the T6 dermatome.

Future developments

Training and maintenance of skills in the technique of PCC is crucial. The learning curve in this procedure is not as steep as that for other pain relief interventional techniques. As the number of centres offering this procedure is very small, the training opportunities are very limited with the risk of this technique becoming extinct. This important issue needs to be addressed by national organizations responsible for training in pain medicine in various countries. CT/MRI-guided technique for PCC has been described and may have some advantages especially in cases with difficult anatomy. This, however, does not seem to be popular. Endoscopic technique of cervical cordotomy has also been recently described. This may have some advantages.

Conclusion

Key learning points

- Cordotomy is a very effective pain relief technique for cancer pain.
- It is relatively safe and a one-off technique.
- Pain relief can last many months.
- Usually there is significant reduction in opioid intake and improved quality of life.
- Careful patient selection and informed consent is important as there can be serious complications, though these are extremely rare in expert hands.

Further reading

Bain E, Hugel H, Sharma M (2013). Percutaneous cervical cordotomy for the management of pain from cancer: A prospective review of 45 cases. *J Palliat Med*, **16**(8), 901–7.

Crul B, Laura BM, van Egmond J, van Dongen RTM (2005). The present role of percutaneous cervical cordotomy for the treatment of cancer pain. *J Headache Pain*, **6**, 24–9.

Ischia S, Luzzani A, Ischia A, Maffezzoli G (1984). Bilateral percutaneous cervical cordotomy: immediate and long-term results in 36 patients with neoplastic disease. *J Neurol Neurosurg Psychiatry*, **47**, 141–7.

Jackson MB, Pounder D, Price C, Matthews AW, Neville E (1999). Percutaneous cervical cordotomy for the control of pain in patients with pleural mesothelioma. *Thorax*, **54**, 238–41.

Lipton S (1968). Percutaneous electrical cordotomy in relief of intractable pain. *BMJ*, **2**, 210–2.

Lipton S (1973). Pain control and the management of advanced malignant disease. *Proc R Soc Med*, **66**, 7–9.

Mesothelioma Framework (2007). Available at: ✆ <http://www.mesothelioma.uk.com/editorim-ages/DOH%20Framework%20for%20Mesothelioma.pdf> (accessed 20 April 2013).

Nagaro T, Kimura S, Arai T (1987). A mechanism of new pain following cordotomy; reference of sensation. *Pain*, **30**, 89–91.

Price C, Pounder D, Jackson M, Rogers P, Neville E (2003). Respiratory function after unilateral percutaneous cervical cordotomy. *J Pain Sympt Manag*, **25**(5), 459–63.

Sluijter M (2002). Technical aspects of radiofrequency. *Pain Pract*, **2**(3), 195–200.

Intrathecal drug delivery for cancer pain

Louise Lynch

Introduction 198
Background knowledge 199
Drugs 201
   Opioids 201
   Local anaesthetic 201
   Clonidine 202
   Ziconotide 202
   Other drugs 202
Patient selection 203
   Life expectancy 203
   Diagnosis 203
   Infection 204
   Bleeding diatheses 204
   Psychiatric and psychological
     problems 204
Types of intrathecal drug delivery
   systems 205
   Subcutaneous ports 205
   Fully implanted ITDD
     systems 205
   Gas-driven constant infusion
     ITDD system 206
   Programmable, battery
     powered, fully implanted
     ITDD systems 207
   Test doses and trials 209
Implant procedure 210
   Potential problems and
     complications 210

Infusion regimens 212
   Opioid-sensitive pain 212
   Opioid-insensitive pain 213
   Bupivacaine, opioid, and
     clonidine mixes 214
   Bupivacaine 215
   Ziconotide 215
Metastatic bone pain case
   discussion 216
   Background 216
   Case discussion 216
Perineal pain case discussion 218
   Background 218
   Case discussion 218
Pelvic pain case discussion 220
   Case discussion 220
Sacral and lumbar nerve root
   compression by tumour case
   discussion 222
   Background 222
   Case discussion 222
Conclusion 224
   Key learning points 224
Further reading 225

Introduction

Intrathecal drug delivery (ITDD) has been an option for the management of persistent cancer pain since the 1980s. The discovery of opioid receptors in the central nervous system was the impetus for early attempts to deliver opioids intraspinally. Approximately 1–2% of patients with cancer suffer inadequate analgesia from conventional medical management; this group particularly may benefit from ITDD. However, there is also some evidence for the use of ITDD in those with non-cancer pain. ITDD is also in common use for the administration of IT baclofen to manage spasticity. This chapter will cover ITDD and the systems available for use. Intracerebroventricular (ICV) mode of delivery of opioid is also well known and effective and can be used in head and neck cancer pain. This chapter is about practicalities rather than theory.

ITDD is without doubt underused in the management of complex cancer pain. The number of patients who would benefit is relatively small, but for some, there is no acceptable or effective alternative. The place of ITDD systems is not just at the very end of life in a hospital/hospice setting, but should be part of an ongoing symptom management strategy well before that point. Space can be made in chemotherapy regimens for pain control implants, whether the ultimate goal is palliative or curative. There is a role, too, in cancer survivors, particularly those with treatment-related pain conditions. The development of multidisciplinary working between surgeons, oncologists, palliative medicine physicians, psychiatrists, psychologists, social workers, chaplaincy, other allied health professionals, *and* pain management specialists means that there is the potential to identify suitable patients early on in their journey.

The aim of the chapter is to describe patient selection parameters, to outline the systems and drugs available, and to discuss drug and patient management options in some detail, including a selection of case studies.

ICV opioid delivery is not discussed, although the party line (from Bandolier) is that it is at least as effective as epidural or subarachnoid therapy in patients with intractable cancer pain. The review on which this is based was published in 1996 and the quality of the base data and the endpoints used probably debatable. There are no recently published studies on ICV opioids since the end of the period covered by the last Cochrane review in November 2004.

Background knowledge

Some science and theory or 'background knowledge' is essential to choose and use equipment and drugs.

The target sites for opioids administered either via the epidural or IT route are pre- and postsynaptic receptors of primary afferent pain neurons in the superficial laminae (I–III) of the spinal cord. The majority are in the substantia gelatinosa—a mass of gelatinous grey matter that lies on the dorsal surface of the dorsal columns. The overall effect of opioids is to depress neurotransmitter release and hyperpolarize neuronal membranes thus making the neuron less responsive to pain signal input. The μ-opioid receptor is linked to presynaptic calcium channels by a G-protein-coupled mechanism. Opioids inhibit this channel, but indirectly and partially (unlike ziconotide which binds directly to it) as not all μ-receptors are linked to calcium channels. With time there is a functional uncoupling of the link resulting in tolerance—this does not happen with ziconotide.

Opioid receptors are widely distributed throughout the central neuraxis and although this is responsible for both serious and intolerable side effects, some of the central effects of opioids have a useful role in pain management.

Opioids and local anaesthetics are the mainstay of therapy but other drugs can be used. The Polyanalgesic Consensus Conferences in 2007 and 2012 have developed algorithms for the choice of drugs and recommendations for maximum IT doses and concentrations. These 'conferences' are a group of invited individuals recognized to be experts in ITDD from all over the world, whose purpose is to consider new evidence as it becomes available and to make recommendations based on both the evidence and their experience as practitioners. See Tables 17.1 and 17.2.

Table 17.1 2012 polyanalgesic algorithm for IT therapies in neuropathic pain

Line 1	Morphine	Ziconotide		Morphine + bupivacaine
Line 2	Hydromorphone	Hydromorphone + bupivacaine or hydromorphone + clonidine		Morphine + clonidine
Line 3	Clonidine	Ziconotide + opioid	Fentanyl	Fentanyl + bupivacaine or fentanyl + clonidine
Line 4	Opioid + clonidine + bupivacaine	Bupivacaine + clonidine		
Line 5	Baclofen			

Reproduced from Timothy R. Deer et al., Licensed content title Polyanalgesic Consensus Conference 2012: Recommendations for the Management of Pain by Intrathecal (Intraspinal) Drug Delivery: Report of an Interdisciplinary Expert Panel, Neuromodulation, Volume 15, Issue 5, pp. 436–64, Copyright © 2012 International Neuromodulation Society, with permission from John Wiley and Sons.

Table 17.2 2012 polyanalgesic algorithm for IT therapies in nociceptive pain

Line 1	Morphine	Hydromorphone	Ziconotide	Fentanyl
Line 2	Morphine + bupivacaine	Ziconotide + opioid	Hydromorphone + bupivacaine	Fentanyl + bupivacaine
Line 3	Opioid + clonidine			Sufentanil
Line 4	Opioid + clonidine + bupivacaine		Sufentanil + bupivacaine or clonidine	
Line 5	Sufentanil + bupivacaine + clonidine			

Reproduced from Timothy R. Deer et al., Licensed content title Polyanalgesic Consensus Conference 2012: Recommendations for the Management of Pain by Intrathecal (Intraspinal) Drug Delivery: Report of an Interdisciplinary Expert Panel, Neuromodulation, Volume 15, Issue 5, pp. 436–64, Copyright © 2012 International Neuromodulation Society, with permission from John Wiley and Sons.

Patients with cancer-related pain and a very limited life expectancy are in a very different clinical situation from a non-cancer chronic pain patient with a 'normal' life expectancy. In the former it may be acceptable to use 'experimental' drugs and those rejected from mainstream practice because of neurotoxicity, e.g. ketamine, when standard infusion regimens have failed to provide adequate analgesia.

It is now clear that CSF does not flow up and down the spinal canal and distribute drugs throughout the neuraxis, but rather oscillates at each level in a series of stacked segmental 'doughnuts' surrounded by peripheral eddy currents. Animal studies have shown that drugs infused at similar rates to those possible with ITDD systems do not distribute beyond the confines of the 'doughnut' adjacent to the catheter port. Even a slow bolus (max. rate 1mL/hour) only serves to distribute the drug more widely within those confines. It is also worth noting that, even though most single lumen spinal catheters are multi-ported, with the intention of distributing drug more widely, the drugs actually only exit the catheter from a single one of these ports.

The pharmacokinetics of drugs in the CSF is a function largely of their fat solubility. Very lipid-soluble opioids are rapidly cleared from the CSF to the epidural fat and blood and in fact can produce a useful systemic effect by this route and very little at all by the IT route. Once in the spinal cord, drug factors (physicochemical and pharmacokinetics) affect the way the drug is partitioned between grey matter, white matter, blood, and fat.

In a pig model developed to map the spread of IT drugs, even the most water-soluble of opioids (morphine) does not distribute within the CSF, but puddles at the end of the catheter.

When implanting a spinal catheter, it is imperative that the catheter tip is either at or slightly above the dermatomal level of the patient's pain AND positioned posteriorly in the spinal canal. The only exception to this is for ziconotide infusion implants when catheter position is not crucial.

Drugs

Morphine and ziconotide are the only drugs licensed for ITDD for pain, but whatever drugs are used should be free from additives and preservatives because of both the potential risk of neurotoxicity and the risk of interaction with CSF proteins, causing precipitates which may block a catheter.

Opioids

Morphine and hydromorphone are used IT whereas fentanyl and diamorphine are commonly used for epidural infusions. Diamorphine can cause pump stall in the Medtronic implanted IT pump and cannot be used with these systems but can be used via external delivery systems. Methadone is neurotoxic and sufentanil is not available in the UK.

It is worth noting that conversion factors between individual opioids and between oral, subcutaneous, intravenous, intranasal, and transdermal opioids have enormous reported variations. There are, no doubt, wide individual patient variations too. Individual centres may have their own conversion charts. These often err on the side of caution. Individual titrations are essential and dose conversion factors can be used as a starting point—more or less drug may be required.

- Morphine is a small water-soluble molecule. A conversion factor of 300mg oral morphine equivalents = 1mg IT morphine is often quoted.
- Hydromorphone is a synthetic lipophilic opioid which is more potent than morphine. The author uses a conversion factor of 200mg oral morphine equivalents = 1mg IT hydromorphone. However, it is generally agreed that hydromorphone is 4–7× more potent than morphine!
- Diamorphine is more lipophilic and more potent than morphine and has been used very successfully both IT and epidurally. It should not be used in the Medtronic Synchromed I or II pumps.
- Fentanyl is a highly lipophilic μ-agonist which is rapidly absorbed into the bloodstream and rapidly cleared from the CSF and spinal cord. It has a very short duration of action and is not currently used in the UK, although appears on the Polyanalgesic Concensus Conference algorithm.
- Opioids, except fentanyl, have been linked to IT granuloma formation, although there are no reports in cancer patients so far. The mechanism appears to be irritation of the dura resulting in the generation of an inflammatory mass and the potential of neurological compromise as a result. In experimental dog models, high drug concentration seems to be a causal factor.

Local anaesthetic

Bupivacaine can be used on its own or in combination with opioids and clonidine. Not all pain is sensitive to opioids, so bupivacaine can have a major role in both short- and long-term pain management. It is available in concentrations of up to 4% (40mg/mL). For other than short-term infusions it is usually more effective to use bolus-based regimens, as otherwise tachyphylaxis and loss of clinical effect occurs. Boluses of only 1mg or 2mg can be effective although up to 20mg can be used—these boluses are infused at a maximum rate of 1mL/hour—i.e. the shortest duration of a 20mg bolus would be 30 minutes—not that fast then! The major problem with using local anaesthetics is the loss of sensation which can (but not invariably) come with use. Motor block and incontinence or urinary retention are more uncommon, unless a pre-existing problem. Patients sometimes feel that they would rather have pain than loss of sensation.

Clonidine

Clonidine is an α_2 adrenoceptor agonist and has a variety of effects including reducing the release of C fibre neurotransmitter levels (e.g. substance P and calcitonin gene-related peptide), reducing preganglionic sympathetic outflow and postsynaptic membranes. It can be effective for neuropathic pain in doses of between 60–1000 micrograms/day. It has a synergistic antinociceptive interaction with other drugs, no tolerance, and may be protective against granuloma formation. It is more stable than other drugs in combination with ziconotide. However, abrupt withdrawal can be fatal and any reduction in dose needs to be gradual.

Ziconotide

Ziconotide is a relatively new drug (approved in 2004–5) and not widely available in the UK—requests for funding for the drug have to be made for each patient to the Specialised Services Individual Funding Request Panel in the UK. Its role in cancer pain management has not been established fully, although the original studies on the drug were promising. It is a synthetic analogue of the ω-conotoxin from a sea snail and blocks presynaptic n-type calcium channels in the superficial laminae (I and II) of the dorsal horn, as mentioned earlier. The molecule is very different from the commonly used IT drugs in that it is relatively big (25 amino acids) and completely ionized. Radiolabelling studies in rats have shown that, unlike the opioids which merely puddle at the catheter port, ziconotide distributes widely through the spinal cord and central nervous system. This means it has both the potential to treat a wide variety of pain conditions from an IT catheter at any level, but also to cause a wide range of side effects. Side effects are common and generally reported as mild to moderate and transient, although may necessitate the termination of therapy. All will then settle, although this may take some time—weeks to months. The top 10 are dizziness (53%), headache (35%), nystagmus (30%), somnolence (27%), memory impairment (22%), abnormal gait (21%), nausea (51%), vomiting (19%), constipation (19%), and fever (20%). Ziconotide is specifically contraindicated in patients having IT chemotherapy and those with a clinically defined psychosis. Caution must be used too in depressive illnesses, as it may also exacerbate symptoms to intolerable levels.

Other drugs

Other drugs can be used, but are not in mainstream practice in the UK. Methadone and ketamine are neurotoxic, but may still have a role in the terminal cancer patient if other drugs have proved insufficient.

There are drugs which have been proven to be safe for IT use, but the efficacy for use in chronic pain has not been established. These include gabapentin, baclofen, octreotide, and ropivacaine.

The drugs that have demonstrated neurotoxicity and are not recommended for use (except in special cases) include:
- Opioids (pethidine, methadone, and tramadol)
- Local anaesthetic (tetracaine)
- Adrenergic agonist (dexmedetomidine)
- NMDA antagonists (ketamine)
- Non-opioids (droperidol, midazolam, methylprednisolone, and ondansetron).

Patient selection

Both the Polyanalgesic Consensus Conference and the British Pain Society have recommendations and advice regarding patient selection for ITDD systems. Local expertise, available resources, and referral practice have a huge influence. It is sometimes possible to identify prospective patients early on in their oncology management—either because of the nature of their disease or from difficulties tolerating analgesics.

ITDD systems are effective for pain below the diaphragm—it is possible to site catheters higher than this, to cover chest and arm and shoulder pain, but drug doses are effectively limited by cardiorespiratory side effects. Ziconotide is the exception as it can be used to manage pain of almost any origin from an implanted ITDD system—limiting factors are the necessarily slow titration regimen and side effect profile.

Life expectancy

If death is imminent then a fully implanted system is unfeasible, but a spinal catheter connected to an external pump is an option.

If death is not imminent then fully implanted systems are an option, although an estimated life expectancy of 3 months is often quoted as a cut-off point. An estimated life expectancy of >3 months is often quoted as a cut-off for using a fully implanted ITDD system. There are no absolutes, but as the titration phase for ziconotide can take several months, estimated life expectancy needs to be substantially more than this.

Diagnosis

It may seem obvious that a proper diagnosis is mandatory and that any investigative work or referral to surgeons or other specialists should be done before an ITDD implant. The treatment of the pain is the treatment of the cause of the pain, unless that is not possible. It is still not uncommon to uncover a treatable cause, e.g. gut ischaemia or bowel strictures, as a cause of abdominal pain. Metastatic bone disease may still be amenable to radiotherapy or a definitive orthopaedic procedure. There is often a treatment-related flare of pain for 2 weeks or so after radiotherapy and any decision regarding ITDD is best left until after this period. Spinal disease is worth an opinion from a spinal or neurosurgeon. Vertebroplasty or spinal fusion or stabilization might be options.

A spinal MRI scan is a prerequisite to an implanted ITDD system, if only to illustrate and describe spinal anatomy and to use as a baseline if abnormal neurological symptoms develop subsequently. Asymptomatic multilevel impending cord compression is not uncommon in patients with advanced cancer.

Chemotherapy regimens can usually be adjusted to accommodate the period of time required to implant a pump and for a reasonable healing period afterwards.

Infection

Infection is a relative contraindication. Systemic infection is an absolute contraindication. Sometimes a low-grade chronic infection in the pelvis with recurrent progressive cervical cancer, for example, can be managed with antibiotics to allow an implant or catheter. Progressive cancer is often associated with a high CRP and although an infection screen should be performed it may be safe to proceed.

Bleeding diatheses

Bleeding diatheses are another absolute contraindication, but it may be possible to manage anticoagulated patients according to local haematology protocols.

Psychiatric and psychological problems

Psychiatric and psychological problems are sometimes entirely masked by high doses of opioids and neuropathic pain medication. Psychosis is a contraindication for ziconotide, but it otherwise seems harsh to deny a cancer pain patient an effective treatment for pain on psychological or psychiatric grounds—they are naturally often more difficult to manage after implant though.

Patients often have very strong opinions about drug delivery systems and about what they will and will not be prepared to accept. Separate information sessions led by specialist nurses are helpful for all patients. Some patients are not prepared to make additional trips to a regional centre for reprogramming or refills and for some this may be just a couple of miles from their home. Willingness to attend has to be established well before implant. Distance can be a logistical problem around the time of death when a refill at a patient's home or hospice bed may be necessary. Some centres are well equipped in terms of trained manpower to deliver this and others do not have the resources.

Types of intrathecal drug delivery systems

The simplest systems involve IT catheters attached to an external infusion pump. The advantage of these is that they can be sited without imaging at the patient's bedside using standard equipment available in most anaesthetic departments and high volumes of drugs can be delivered. The disadvantages include the necessity of trained staff, a hospital or hospice bed, likelihood of catheter misplacement, and high infection rates.

Tunnelling the catheter reduces infection rates and using catheter fixing devices makes their position more secure. Patients may be able to be nursed at home if trained staff is available.

Subcutaneous ports

These 'portacath' type systems have a metallic reservoir component with a silicone septum. A spinal catheter can be attached to the reservoir. They are more secure and have lower infection rates than tunnelled catheters.

Fully implanted ITDD systems

Fully implanted ITDD systems are of two types—either fixed rate gas driven or variable rate battery powered.

Codman manufacture the gas driven pump and Medtronic and Flowonix the two variable rate pumps on the market in the UK. A third variable rate pump, the Medstream from Codman, was previously available.

Each manufacturer has intrathecal catheters to fit their pumps. These are single-lumen, multi-ported and non-kinking, even when tied in a knot. Anchors are provided to fix the catheter to the spinal ligaments and are available in one- or two-piece units with connectors, for ease of tunnelling. The Medtronic Ascenda™ (Figure 17.1) and the Flowonix catheter (Figure 17.2) are shown.

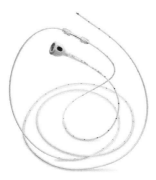

Figure 17.1 Medtronic Ascenda™ catheter. Image courtesy of Medtronic, Inc. Copyright © Medtronic. Inc. 2013.

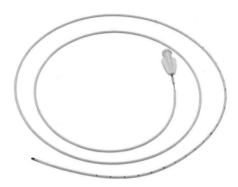

Figure 17.2 Flowonix catheter. Image courtesy of Flowonix Medical Inc., www.flowonix.com, Copyright © 2013 Flowonix Medical Inc.

Gas-driven constant infusion ITDD system

The ARCHIMEDES® is a gas-driven constant flow pump manufactured by Codman (Johnson & Johnson). It is a circular titanium pump with two access ports—a central refill port and a peripheral catheter access port. There is an inner chamber containing infusate, which leaves through a filter and flow restrictor to the spinal catheter, and an outer chamber containing propellant. The pump has a constant infusion rate, so in order to change the amount of drug delivered, the concentration of the infusate has to be changed. There is no way of stopping the pump other than by emptying it. The pump is available in reservoir volumes of 20mL, 35mL, 40mL, 50mL, and 60mL and flow rates of 0.5mL, 0.8mL, 1.0mL, 1.3mL, 1.5mL, 2.0mL, and 3.0mL/day. The lifespan of the pump is around 10 years. It is suitable for patients with stable pain conditions and as such, would have a role in the management of cancer survivors.

Programmable, battery powered, fully implanted ITDD systems

The Synchromed® II (Figure 17.3) is a programmable titanium battery powered pump manufactured by Medtronic. It has a diameter of slightly less than 9cm and weighs around 170g when empty and 200g when full—the reservoir chamber will hold either 20mL or 40mL. There is a bacterial filter and central and side access ports. The central port accesses the reservoir chamber and the side port gives direct access to the spinal catheter. It is possible to access the CSF through this port, either for sampling in cases of possible infection or for direct bolusing of drugs—analgesics or antibiotics. The minimum flow rate is 0.048mL/day and the maximum is 1.0mL/hr. The pump can be programmed to deliver simple continuous infusions or complex variable rate infusions.

A recent arrival in the UK is the Prometra by Flowonix (Figure 17.4). The pump has a 20mL reservoir and employs a valve-gated mechanism to pump the infusate rather the peristaltic system using motors and rota arms employed by the Synchromed II. This is designed to produce a precise controlled drug flow. It is possible to stop the pump completely (unlike the Synchromed II) and flow rates up to 28mL/day can be achieved. Battery life is estimated at 10 years with a flow rate of 0.25mL/day. It may be possible to use diamorphine with this pump.

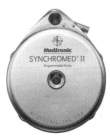

Figure 17.3 Synchromed® battery powered pump. Image courtesy of Medtronic, Inc. Copyright © Medtronic. Inc. 2013.

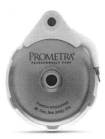

Figure 17.4 Flowonix Prometra intrathecal infusion pump figure source note: Image courtesy of Flowonix Medical Inc., www.flowonix.com, Copyright © 2013 Flowonix Medical Inc.

There is a separate programming unit called the N'Vision® (Figure 17.5). Medtronic are the only manufacturer to offer a patient therapy manager 'PTM' (Figure 17.6). This is a slave unit to the pump itself which can be programmed via the N'Vision®, to enable bolusing on demand according to pre-set parameters of dose, duration of infusion, lock-out interval, and maximum number of activations per 24 hours. This is a major advantage in the management of fluctuating progressive cancer-related pain. There are arguments for the use of bolus-based regimens in a much wider context as pain relief is often managed more effectively when required without resorting to oral drugs and their side effects. There is less tolerance and tachyphylaxis to opioids and bupivacaine and it is certainly possible theoretically that there would be less likelihood of granulomas developing with a low-background, intermittent bolus regimen, than a high-background, infusion-based one. The disadvantage is that bolus-based regimens have the potential to reduce time between refills (although not necessarily so) and can substantially reduce battery life. Battery life is estimated at 6–7 years with 'normal' usage, but can be much less than a year in a big bolus-based regimen—although these are usually the patients towards the end of their life, so it is not a practical problem.

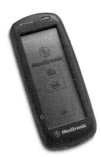

Figure 17.5 N'Vision® to programme pump. Image courtesy of Medtronic, Inc. Copyright © Medtronic. Inc. 2013.

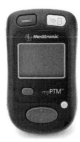

Figure 17.6 Patient therapy manager. Image courtesy of Medtronic, Inc. Copyright © Medtronic. Inc. 2013.

Test doses and trials

For other than systems using external pumps, some form of test dose or trial is recommended. One has to be practical here though and sometimes it is not feasible for a variety of reasons—transfer from another centre and children are examples. The issues are different for patients with progressive cancer-related pain from those with chronic non-cancer pain—they are arguably the same for cancer pain survivors.

An ideal trial would replicate the features of the fully implanted system. This is achievable for straightforward simple infusions but not for the more complex, often bolus-based regimens used for progressive fluctuating cancer-related pain.

I aim to trial a single bolus for patients with cancer-related pain. This may be a single drug or a mixture. From the bolus I hope to get an idea of whether or not the pain is opioid sensitive, and what sort of doses are going to be needed. For example, if a 0.5mg bolus of hydromorphone gives good quality pain relief for 12 hours then I am confident that the pain is opioid sensitive and that maybe 1mg/day would be a good starting background infusion. I also know whether the bolus has had any adverse effects, which would indicate caution particularly if we are going to use a bolus-based regimen.

If I have used a mix of hydromorphone, clonidine, and bupivacaine and only 2–4 hours of adequate analgesia is reported, then either I have used an insufficient dose of opioid or the pain is partially sensitive to it.

I use a dose conversion of 1mg IT hydromorphone being approximately equivalent to 200mg of oral morphine equivalents. This gives a 24-hour dose estimate. I then divide by 2 for a 12-hour dose to use for a bolus.

For example, for a patient on 2000mg oral morphine equivalents the 24-hour IT dose of hydromorphone would be 10mg and the bolus dose 5mg. For a patient on 40mg oral morphine equivalents the 24-hour IT dose would be 0.2mg and the bolus 0.1mg.

The bolus dose of clonidine is 15–30 micrograms and of bupivacaine from 1–2mg, although very occasionally is higher than this.

Implant procedure

To implant an IT pump a full theatre set-up with anaesthetist is mandatory.

Antibiotic cover will vary according to local guidelines—for our centre a single shot of teicoplanin and 2mg/kg of gentamicin is the current recommendation.

My personal preference is to perform implants using local anaesthesia and minimal sedation.

As mentioned previously it is essential to position the catheter dorsally within the spinal canal and to be at either the dermatomal level of the patient's pain or very slightly above.

The pump pocket is usually either in the right or left iliac fossa, although if these sites are already occupied to stomas etc. then either upper quadrant works as well. It is worth checking with oncology preoperatively whether or not further radiotherapy may be an option and if so, are there any particular sites to be avoided.

The patient is of course, fasted preoperatively and will be a bit 'on the dry side' in terms of hydration. To minimize the effects of the procedure (I use a bolus of IT bupivacaine for the pump implant), the effects of the other IT drugs and protect against the risk of post-dural puncture headache, it is important to rehydrate the patient with IV fluids during surgery and maintain hydration afterwards. An IV infusion of at least 24–48 hours may be required. CSF lost during the procedure can be replaced with normal saline during it—care is required though as unpleasant neuropathic pain will result from energetic use of cold saline and take some time to resolve.

The pump itself is emptied of the fluid in the reservoir chamber and filled with the chosen infusate prior to placing in the prepared pocket. Ideally both a priming bolus and an additional IT bolus are initiated when the pump is connected to the spinal catheter to ensure that the patient is free from their normal cancer-related pain in the recovery period. This is also a time to assess the effect of this IT bolus and to make adjustments to the proposed IT regimen accordingly.

Patients with cancer pain would usually need a few days postoperatively to both recover from the procedure and to make adjustments to their pump and other drug requirements. Immediately postoperatively opioid requirements can be halved and then halved again every 72 hours. Patients will, of course, need close monitoring and sometimes this process is more or less rapid. Sometimes relief of pain from one site will unmask a previously unknown problem at another.

Potential problems and complications

Problems are related to the equipment and its component parts and to the drug/s infused. Patients with cancer-related pain can of course have recurrence or progression of their disease and new symptoms need assessing with this in mind.

Wound infections, pump pocket infections, infection tracking back along the catheter, and meningitis are all possible. The last two are irretrievable in terms of salvaging the system, which must be removed as an emergency procedure. The system will be at risk during episodes of bacteraemia and septicaemia and so any such episodes should be treated aggressively, even during terminal care.

Bleeding around surgical sites is always possible and there is a risk of intraspinal haematoma.

There is the potential for CSF leak, seroma formation, and post-dural puncture headache. Most headaches will resolve with hydration, caffeine, and bed rest, but if there is CSF hypotension, there is the risk of a sub-dural haematoma. If the headache persists and is associated with nausea and vomiting or neurology changes then a CT scan is required. Unlike in anaesthetic practice where epidural blood patches are used quite happily, there would have to be a much greater risk of infection in a patient with a newly implanted pump.

Catheters can become displaced or occluded.

Gear shaft wear and motor stall are rare in the UK and most of Europe, but more common in the US and Germany.

IT granulomas commonly present with deterioration in pain control, new pain, and new neurological symptoms and signs. None has yet been reported in cancer pain patients, but they would have to be in the differential diagnosis and radiologists should be aware that the appearance of a granuloma can mimic abscess or tumour. Management of an identified granuloma may include cessation of opioid infusion and replacement with saline, resiting of the catheter or surgical removal of the granuloma.

Peripheral oedema can occur in those with a predisposition to develop it and it can be markedly exacerbated in those who have it already. The mechanism is unknown but opioids have both an effect on antidiuretic hormone levels and on the sympathetic nervous system.

Opioids can cause hormonal changes by inducing hypogonadotropic hypogonadism and thus lower levels of oestrogen or testosterone. ITDD does not prevent this altogether but as the mechanism is central, one would expect the incidence and severity to be lower—hormone replacement is certainly possible, if necessary.

Hyperalgesia is another central effect of opioids and may be important in patients on high doses of oral/SC/transdermal/IV opioids. It could explain reduced pain levels when oral drugs are weaned and lead to some confusion when trying to calculate IT doses.

Drowsiness is *not* a usual associated feature of ITDD systems containing opioids, clonidine, and bupivacaine. Another cause must be sought.

Infusion regimens

Several recommendations have been made for minimizing the potential neurotoxicity of infused drugs:

- Minimizing local concentrations of drugs against neural tissue by appropriate catheter placement
- High flow rates
- Using the lowest drug concentration possible and more complex dosing regimens
- Demand or activity-based dosing
- Variable flow rates
- Intermittent bolus delivery.

The Polyanalgesic Consensus Conference in 2012 produced recommendations for maximum intrathecal doses and concentrations. See Table 17.3.

Table 17.3 Concentrations and doses of IT agents by the Polyanalgesic Consensus Panellists 2012

Drug	Maximum concentration	Maximum dose per day
Morphine	20mg/mL	15mg
Hydromorphone	15mg/mL	10mg
Fentanyl	10mg/mL	No known upper limit
Sufentanil	5mg/mL	No known upper limit
Bupivacaine	30mg/mL	10mg
Clonidine	1000 micrograms/mL	40–600 micrograms/day
Ziconotide	100 micrograms/mL	19.2 micrograms/day

Reproduced from Timothy R. Deer et al., Licensed content title Polyanalgesic Consensus Conference 2012: Recommendations for the Management of Pain by Intrathecal (Intraspinal) Drug Delivery: Report of an Interdisciplinary Expert Panel, *Neuromodulation*, Volume 15, Issue 5, pp. 436–64, Copyright © 2012 International Neuromodulation Society, with permission from John Wiley and Sons.

The aims and objectives of managing a patient with progressive cancer-related pain are to achieve pain control within the shortest period of time to maximize quality of life for the remainder of the patient's life. Sometimes it is both appropriate and acceptable to relax some of the theoretical constraints of ITDD in non-cancer patients and in selected cases to consider other drugs; see case discussions later in chapter.

Opioid-sensitive pain

We use hydromorphone in our institution, rather than morphine. The reasons for this are largely historical as we previously used diamorphine and when we had to change this, the natural choice was hydromorphone with its more similar pharmacokinetics. We have used concentrations of 1–10mg/mL. If pain is very opioid sensitive, for example, metastatic bone pain, then simple background infusions of opioid can be very effective. There will be valuable information from the IT test dose. If this has been effective for the predicted 12 hours then a 24-hour infusion of double this dose is a good starting point. If it has been effective for >24 hours then probably much less will be sufficient. If <12 hours but still good quality then more is likely to be needed. If, however, the bolus has given poor quality analgesia for <12 hours then another regimen should be considered.

Background dose increases may be required over time and 25–30% increases can cover this. If these are requested on a regular basis, then it is probably appropriate to go onto a bolus-based regimen with a lower background infusion—thus delivering potentially the same dose of opioid but in a different format. Sometimes much less opioid is actually required. The addition of clonidine may improve analgesia.

Loss of previously good pain control necessitates reassessment of the clinical situation as well as pump and catheter checks. Disease progression must be excluded, along with pump malfunction and catheter blockage.

In the event of disease progression an opioid-bolus-based regimen may be effective but the addition of bupivacaine may helpful at this point—initially in low doses or 1mg or 2mg per bolus.

The maximum interval between pump refills is 12 weeks. Opioids are stable in solution up to this time, which is also true for mixes of opioids with clonidine and bupivacaine. This would be very acceptable for someone with stable disease. Concentrations of opioid can be chosen to accommodate refill intervals within the consensus guidelines above. For example, a patient managed on a background infusion rate of 0.3mg hydromorphone/day could have an infusate of 1mg/mL or 40mg hydromorphone in 40mL water. This will last for 133 days and refills can be every 3 months and there is also some scope for increasing the dose before the refill date is due if necessary. For a patient on 1mg/day, a concentration of 3mg/mL (120mg in 40mL) would be acceptable and so on.

For patients on a bolus-based regime, it is slightly more complicated to calculate the refill date as the pump will initially give a date based on the background rate set and maximum usage of the boluses available. Most patients with stable disease will have similarly stable bolus usage, but there must still be some flexibility with additional drug available if required. For example, if a patient uses two boluses per day there still should be the flexibility for a third and possibly a fourth, but as this is not going to happen on a daily basis, the refill date can still be after the calculated alarm date given when the pump is reprogrammed with the refill. For example if the alarm date is 6 June initially but fewer boluses than the maximum are actually used, the alarm date will be continually reset to a later date. The PTM gives the estimated date of the pump alarm or refill in big letters on the start-up screen.

Opioid-insensitive pain

Some patients have pain either not at all sensitive to opioids or with limited sensitivity. Often they present on huge doses of a variety of opioids given by a variety of routes and rarely on none at all. Some cases of nerve root compression and perineal pain secondary to tumour breakdown are illustrative examples. Options then are either to use a local anaesthetic mix with opioid and clonidine or pure local anaesthetic or consider ziconotide. Each of these options is considered as follows.

Bupivacaine, opioid, and clonidine mixes

These mixes are stable with the commonly used IT opioids. They are effective for pain below the diaphragm, i.e. with an IT catheter placed below T6—above this level the side effects of bradycardia and hypotension limit effective use of the drugs. The advantage of a drug mix is that there is often a synergistic effect on pain and lower doses of local anaesthetic can be used to greater effect on pain, whilst minimizing the side effects of the local. Many patients do not like numbness and would prefer pain rather than an abnormal sensation. This is the same for ziconotide which may relieve the pain of a peripheral neuropathy, but the underlying abnormal neuropathy remains.

When calculating mixes, it is useful to the clinician to be aware of the concentrations of drugs available to the hospital pharmacy that are making up the syringes for refill, as this will affect the final concentration of bupivacaine. The prescription must also be clear—if you want 5mg/mL of bupivacaine in your syringe it should be clear that you need 200mg in 40mL and that you do not want the diluent to be 0.5% bupivacaine or there is a strong chance that after the hydromorphone and clonidine have been added, the syringe will be filled to the final volume of 40mL with it, which may reduce the concentration down to 2.5mg/mL. Pharmacies have an online list of their stock. Our pharmacy uses 50mg/mL hydromorphone, 2mg/mL clonidine (but beware 150 micrograms/mL also available!) and has 4% (40mg/mL) bupivacaine. Unless the syringe has been requested as pure 4% bupivacaine there is likely to be much less in it. A mix containing 10mg/mL hydromorphone and 120 micrograms/mL clonidine can only have a maximum of just less than 30mg/mL, i.e. <3% bupivacaine if the remainder of the syringe is filled with 4% once the other drugs are added.

Given the constraints mentioned, syringes can contain mixes of 1–10mg/mL hydromorphone, 60–480 micrograms/mL clonidine, and up to 40mg/mL bupivacaine. Patients using drug mixes are generally more complex than those on simple opioid background infusions and a refill and review interval of 4–5 weeks is useful. I tend to calculate a mix which will use 1mL of infusate per day.

For example, a patient on 800mg/day oral morphine equivalents, who has half an IT test dose of 2mg hydromorphone with 30 micrograms clonidine and 2mg of bupivacaine and had 4–6 hours of reasonable quality pain relief, one might choose a mix of 5mg/mL hydromorphone with 120 micrograms/mL clonidine and 10mg/mL bupivacaine and start with a low background infusion rate of 1mg hydromorphone/day and a bolus of 0.5mg hydromorphone with 12 micrograms clonidine and 1mg bupivacaine, which can be used up to eight times per day. If this bolus is insufficient it can be increased to 1mg hydromorphone with 24 micrograms clonidine and 2mg bupivacaine up to 4 times per day.

The ratios of drugs can only be changed at refills, of course.

The maximum drug concentrations we currently use are 10mg/mL hydromorphone with 120–480 micrograms/mL clonidine and 3% bupivacaine. The maximum bolus is 5mg hydromorphone with 60–240 micrograms clonidine and 15mg bupivacaine over 30 minutes.

If using a bolus-based regimen, the ultimate goal is obviously to achieve good quality 'as required' pain control. As such, it is important to find a good bolus dose and to enable the patient to use these top-ups as frequently as they need them. Initially patients tend to use boluses as often as they can to ensure good pain relief. Once they have confidence that the bolus is effective, then the frequency of use often reduces dramatically—for example, a bolus used hourly may be saved for only two or three times a day. Lock-out settings should be set, not to restrict bolus use, but to facilitate achieving good pain control. A 20-minute lock-out setting is thus much kinder than a 4-hour one. Similarly, an unrestricted number of potential boluses per day may enable initial 'overuse', but the price for this is more frequent trips to hospital for refills. A good general rule is to set a short lock-out interval and a generous number of activations and let the patient self-regulate their pain.

Bupivacaine

Pure bupivacaine can be used; 4% (40mg/mL) is available. I have found it particularly useful for patients with perineal pain when I have passed a retrograde catheter to the bottom of the dural sac at S2. Boluses here cause minimum side effects when compared with higher sipinal levels and seem much better tolerated.

Ziconotide

Ziconotide is an option for non-opioid sensitive pain and for pain above the diaphragm, but the titration regimen needs to be slow and can take several months, so time is needed. It is an expensive drug (although actually not much more so than some of the standard hydromorphone mixes) and many regions demand individual applications for funding, which results in yet more delay.

Creatine kinase levels may rise during therapy. A baseline level must be taken prior to starting an infusion and then at intervals throughout. If there is a progressive rise, there is a risk of myopathy and rhabdomyolysis and the infusion must be stopped. It is safe to stop ziconotide and the CSF level will drop to 5% of its infusion level in 24 hours after discontinuing treatment.

The drug adsorbs onto pump components, so it is recommended that the pump is washed with several syringes of the drug before use. The first refill has to be 14 days after implant for the same reason. Subsequent refills have to be at 40 days if diluted ziconotide is used and every 84 days for the 'neat' solution, depending on dose.

The initial infusion rate in 2.4 micrograms/day. The recommendation is that dose increases of no more than 2.4 micrograms/day are made no more than two or three times/week. The maximum recommended dose is 19.2 micrograms/day. There is obviously a trade-off between 'rapid' dose increases and side effects and a much slower titration of 1.2 micrograms every 2 weeks is both better tolerated and therefore more successful.

Ziconotide can be used as part of a drug mix but this reduces drug stability, particularly when more than two drugs are used. Refills have to be every 4 weeks with hydromorphone and every 2 weeks if bupivacaine is used in addition.

Metastatic bone pain case discussion

Background

Bone pain is often very opioid sensitive and a simple background infusion of a relatively low dose of opioid may be sufficient.

The following case discussion serves to illustrate the very individual nature of each patient's pain and that initial strategies may need to change to manage new problems as they arise.

Case discussion

The 65-year-old patient was referred with a 10-year history of breast cancer and pelvic metastases. She had had a mastectomy and axillary clearance and radiotherapy.

After 8 years' disease free she presented to her GP with hip pain and was subsequently found to have localized pelvic bone metastases in unilateral ilium and acetabulum.

These were managed with radiotherapy, but pain continued and sensitivity to even small doses of opioids prompted pain clinic referral for a 'nerve block'.

A sacroiliac joint injection was 30% effective for a couple of weeks and a hip joint injection was almost 100% effective but for only 2 weeks.

She was then referred for a specialist orthopaedic opinion regarding the feasibility of a hemi-arthroplasty. This was judged to not be possible.

Unfortunately she was not able to tolerate analgesic medication without side effects of nausea, dizziness, and somnolence. She was a very anxious lady and easily distressed on minimal provocation, although seemingly unaware of the implications of progressive nature of her disease.

After many weeks of discussion, she was listed for an IT test dose. This was postponed on the first occasion because of nausea and dizziness on fasting. An intravenous infusion of glucose-saline a couple of hours preprocedure seemed to settle these symptoms the following week and 0.1mg hydromorphone gave excellent analgesia for approximately 36 hours.

The IT pump was implanted uneventfully with the catheter tip at T12 and a starting infusion mix of 1mg/mL hydromorphone. The background rate was set at 0.1mg after a starting bolus of 0.1mg in theatre.

Once home and mobilizing it became clear that this was insufficient and it was titrated up to between 0.26–0.32mg/day over the next 2 months and thereafter oscillated between those values for the next 3 years.

Minimal increases and decreases were made at just about every 3 monthly refill, at the patient's request. She, however, was able to enjoy a completely 'normal' life at home with her new grandchildren and able to travel to the south of France on family holidays.

Prior to pump implant she had been only able to mobilize with sticks in the house and wheelchair when out and had become effectively housebound.

We received a call out of the blue with a story of the pump no longer working and reviewed the following day in clinic. On assessment she had obvious loss of weight from her upper body, but marked oedema from the waist down.

Oncology assessment then revealed extensive pelvic and lumbar spine metastases, along with liver and lung nodules and ascites.

A bolus of 0.1mg hydromorphone given via pump in clinic with good effect and background rate increased to 0.35mg. The patient was not pre-pared to contemplate higher dose or using a PTM.

She then attended on a weekly basis for a small bolus and small increase in background infusion rate until persuaded to trial a PTM. The pump was programmed for the PTM to allow a bolus of 0.1mg over 6 minutes with a lock-out of 2 hours and a maximum activity of four/day. The background infusion rate was increased to run at 1mg/day.

The following week her pain was still not controlled and the bolus was increased to 0.2mg over 12 minutes with a lock-out of 1 hour and maxi-mum activity of 12/day. 0.2mg bolus gave good relief in clinic, but from a telephone call a few days later, she was persuaded to come in for a few days to change the infusion mix and re-establish pain control.

The infusate mix was changed to 5mg/mL hydromorphone + 120 micro-grams/mL clonidine and 5mg/mL bupivacaine. PTM bolus established by using an incremental bolus via the single bolus function on the N'Vision® programmer starting at 0.2mg hydromorphone and increased in 0.2mg increments to 0.8mg. Bolus then set at 1.0mg hydromorphone + 24 micro-grams clonidine + 1.0mg bupivacaine to infuse over 12 minutes with a back-ground rate of 2mg hydromorphone/day. The lockout interval was left at 60 minutes and maximum number of activations at eight/day.

She was discharged home again after 48 hours with her pain well-controlled.

She then attended every 4 weeks for review and pump refills. No further changes were made. She went on to develop a deep vein thrombosis and pulmonary embolus resulting in anticoagulation with warfarin. Increasing oedema around abdomen and pump led to leakage of oedema fluid for several days after each refill but no infection. She eventually died peacefully in a hospice near her home.

Perineal pain case discussion

Background

Perineal pain secondary to recurrent or progressive cancer, commonly of cervix, anus, or penis, is not always particularly opioid sensitive and is frequently associated with a significant degree of distress, which can limit therapeutic options. It ought to be possible to identify these patients at diagnosis of disease recurrence via oncology MDT meetings and early referral means that whatever option is selected can be a cold elective event, rather than a crisis. A retrograde catheter passed to the bottom of the dural sac at around S2 will be both maximally effective and limit the side effects of local anaesthetic at higher levels *but* obviously will not cover pain above S2—if there is a likelihood of the tumour rising out of the pelvis and involving the area of the T12 dermatome, then the catheter is better placed at T12.

Case discussion

A man in his early 40s with penile cancer and local recurrence was referred with severe incapacitating perineal pain, which had developed over the period of a few weeks and was partially opioid responsive.

He was referred to the pain clinic for a nerve block.

He had an IT test dose with 0.6mL of heavy bupivacaine 0.5%, which was completely effective for 2 hours. This was followed by 0.6mL of IT phenol the following day with good effect.

Unfortunately the pain returned immediately after discharge home and he returned for a repeat phenol block. This reproduced his previous pain relief but only for 7 days. One final phenol block was equally effective.

An IT pump was then implanted with a retrograde catheter placed at S2. A mix of 1mg/mL hydromorphone with 120 micrograms/mL clonidine and 5mg/mL bupivacaine was chosen first of all as he was then taking 80mg twice daily slow release morphine with morphine sulfate solution 10mg up to four times a day. A bolus-based regimen was trialled to start with, with a background infusion rate of 0.2mg hydromorphone per day and boluses of 0.2mg hydromorphone (1mg bupivacaine) over 12 minutes up to four times/day.

This worked well and the patient was able to sit comfortably for the first time in several weeks, such that that he missed his first refill—'gone fishing'!

He was also able to resume alpine walking. Fourteen months later he contacted the clinic to report that he had slipped and fallen in Switzerland and his pump had stopped working.

A theatre session with fluoroscopy was booked—on screening the rotor arm of the pump was turning and the pump reservoir contained the volume of drug calculated.

The catheter was accessed by the side port of the pump under X-ray screening and initially aspirated and then radio-opaque dye used to establish catheter position and patency—there was free flow through the catheter tip still at the bottom of the dural sac. A bolus of 1.0mL of 0.5% heavy bupivacaine was given through the side port to re-establish pain control and the catheter then flushed with saline.

The reservoir was then filled with a mix of 2mg/mL hydromorphone with 120 micrograms/mL clonidine and 3% bupivacaine (approximately 25mg/mL). The background infusion was left at 0.2mg hydromorphone/day but the bolus was increased to 0.4mg hydromorphone (5mg bupivacaine) over 12 minutes to be used a maximum of six times/day.

He was referred back to the surgical team for further investigation and found to have significant disease progression. He survived for another 6 months after this and the bolus settings remained at the same dose although the maximum number of activations was increased to 12 in the last couple of weeks.

Pelvic pain case discussion

Case discussion

A 40-year-old lady with pelvic recurrence of cancer of the cervix and associated pelvic and groin pain. She was admitted to one of the inpatient wards for pain control and underwent a fairly rapid opioid titration resulting in profound drowsiness such that she was unrousable on two initial attempted consultations.

She was eventually assessed when awake as an outpatient and went on to have a caudal epidural before an IT test dose. She was on 100mg oral morphine equivalents per 24 hours and had a test dose of 0.3mg hydromorphone + 30 micrograms clonidine + 1mg bupivacaine, which gave 24 hours of good quality pain relief. She went to have a pump implanted 4 weeks later.

Initial mix = 40mg hydromorphone + 4.8mg clonidine to 40mL with 0.5% bupivacaine. The background rate was set at 0.5mg hydromorphone/day with a bolus of 0.1mg hydromorphone + 12 micrograms clonidine + 0.5mg bupivacaine over 6 minutes with a lockout of 2 hours and a maximum of four activations a day.

Pain was well managed on this regimen and all opioids were stopped with an improvement in conscious level.

After 4 months she mentioned a painful cold foot with dry black toes. She remained a heavy smoker during her time with us. A vascular surgery referral was made and interventions then commenced with revascularization procedures to start with and then amputations—initially of individual toes and then the forefoot.

During this time additional analgesia was required although the original pelvic and groin pain remained well controlled.

Initially the background infusion was left at 0.5mg/day of hydromorphone and the bolus was increased from 0.1mg hydromorphone (0.5mg bupivacaine) to 0.4mg hydromorphone (2mg bupivacaine).

2mg bupivacaine gave good quality analgesia for 3–4 hours. The patient, however, did not like the numbness accompanying the analgesia and so we tried increasing the duration of the bolus to 20 and then 30 minutes to minimize this. Boluses were being required up to eight times a day.

Total daily doses at that time were approximately 3mg of hydromorphone and 15mg of bupivacaine.

Pain relief was good using a low background bolus-based regimen, but the patient was not keen still on the inevitable side effects of the local anaesthetic, so we then went on to trial a higher background infusion rate.

The infusion mix was then changed to 200mg bupivacaine (5mg/mL) and 4.8mg clonidine (120 micrograms/mL) to 40mL with 4% bupivacaine giving a local anaesthetic concentration of approximately 33mg/mL.

The background infusion was reset to 3mg hydromorphone and 20mg bupivacaine per day with a bolus facility of 0.3mg hydromorphone and 2mg bupivacaine over 20 minutes with 8 potential boluses per day. The background was then increased further to 5mg hydromorphone and 33mg bupivacaine, then 8/53, then 10/66 and ultimately 12/78 over 24 hours with unchanged bolus settings.

Additional oral oxycodone MR was added by the surgical team with OxyNorm® to be used instead of the PTM boluses up to doses of 20mg twice daily OxyContin® and 5mg 4-hourly of OxyNorm®.

The increased background infusion did provide additional pain control without the intermittent changes in sensation disliked by the patient, but boluses were still required in addition to control fluctuations in pain. The oral opioid produced drowsiness and confusion without pain control and was discontinued.

Overall the trial of using the background infusion only to control the additional ischaemic pain was deemed a failure and the background infusion was reduced over a period of 2 weeks to its previous setting of 0.5mg hydromorphone and 3.3mg bupivacaine per day.

These settings were unchanged for the rest of her life and refills were every 4 to 5 weeks.

Four weeks before death the edge of the pump started to erode through the skin. This was associated with progressive cachexia and the patient was extremely thin. We decided to keep skin edges clean and to use occlusive dressings, rather than to either remove the whole system, or to partially externalize the pump. This fortunately was sufficient and there was no infection to necessitate removal of the system.

Information from the pump manufacturer (Medtronic), at the time, is that the flow rate of the pump will vary with body temperature in a linear fashion. Flow rate will be expected to be approximately 20% less at 21°C than at normal body temperature. It would have been necessary to increase the programmed flow rate accordingly if we had decided to externalize the pump.

Sacral and lumbar nerve root compression by tumour case discussion

Background

These patients are often on huge amounts of opioids prior to referral. It is important to make sure that all treatment options have been explored and in particular a specialist spinal surgery opinion sought and recent MRI obtained both to describe anatomy and rule out cord or cauda equina compression. A reasonable estimate of life expectancy is useful too, as in cases of unilateral nerve root compression and limited life expectancy; cordotomy may be a good option.

Case discussion

A man in his early 40s with a diagnosis of metastatic rectal cancer was referred with a lumbar metastasis compressing his right L5 nerve root and resulting in leg pain. A spinal surgery opinion had been sought prior to referral and surgical decompression not deemed feasible. At the time of presentation he had small volume lung and liver metastases with no change in size over the last 6 months and the view of his oncology team was that his life expectancy might be up to 5 years. He had been alternating several weeks bed-bound in the hospice with time at home with a substantial amount of input from his local GP and district nurses. He was taking in total more than 5g of oral morphine equivalents per day. Flare-ups of pain occurred frequently throughout the day and were managed with escalating doses of opioid until loss of consciousness. Neuropathic pain drugs had had a useful effect early on including ketamine.

The IT test dose had 5mg hydromorphone, 5mg bupivacaine and 30 micrograms clonidine and was completely effective for 4 hours. An IT pump was implanted and the mix chosen comprised 10mg/mL hydromorphone with 240 micrograms/mL clonidine and 4% bupivacaine (27mg/mL final concentration). The background infusion set at 5mg hydromorphone/day and the bolus set at 2mg hydromorphone (5.4mg bupivacaine) over 12 minutes. This was given with the priming bolus in theatre during pump implant and not effective at all. The bolus was repeated immediately with reasonable effect and the bolus reset to 4mg hydromorphone (11mg bupivacaine) over 24 minutes with a lockout of 2 hours and a maximum activity of eight times per day. The bolus was well tolerated with no numbness or motor weakness. Prior to discharge it was increased to maximum deliverable of 5mg hydromorphone (13mg bupivacaine and 120 micrograms clonidine) over 30 minutes. The lockout was reduced to 60 minutes and the maximum activity increased to 12 times per day.

For the first month after implant he was using the PTM approximately eight times per day, but then had a period of 6 months of only a couple of boluses per day. Refills were weekly to start and then 3-weekly during this period of stability. He was able to reduce his other opioids to <100mg/day of oral morphine equivalents. Prior to pump implant he had been calling for medical assistance at night from his GP and these calls for 150mg SC diamorphine also stopped, apart from one occasion when neither the patient nor his wife could get the PTM to work. The problem was in fact, flat batteries rather than anything technical, but from then on he was issued with another PTM and advised on stocking up on batteries and changing them before they were completely flat.

He was then very well managed on the bolus-based regimen, but with weekly refills. He died about a year after pump implant.

Conclusion

Key learning points

- ITDD systems have an important role in managing refractory pain related to cancer, particularly for pain below the diaphragm when cordotomy is not an option. Early referral is imperative to maximize the benefits of the technique.
- A number of systems are available and regimens can be based on continuous infusions or low-background, bolus-based regimens.
- Drugs used include opioids, clonidine, bupivacaine, and ziconotide, either alone or in combinations. Complex progressive cancer-related pain below the diaphragm can often be managed effectively with ITDD systems based on bolus-based regimens using mixtures of drugs.
- MRI scanning is usually possible with the systems *in situ*.
- IT catheter tip must be positioned either at or above the dermatomal level of the patient's pain or at the level at which the cancer might be predicted to spread.

Further reading

British Pain Society (2008). *Intrathecal Drug Delivery for the Management of Pain and Spasticity in Adults: Recommendations for Best Clinical Practice*. Available at: ℰ <http://www.britishpainsociety.org/itdd_main.pdf> (accessed 20 April 2013).

Deer TR, Prager J, Levy R, Rathmell J, Buchser E, Burton A, et al. (2012). Polyanalgesic Consensus Conference (2012): recommendations for the management of pain by intrathecal (intraspinal) drug delivery: report of an interdisciplinary expert panel. *Neuromodulation*, **15**, 436–66.

Hester J, Sykes N, Peat S (2012). *Interventional Pain Control in Cancer Pain Management* (see chapters 5–7). Oxford: Oxford University Press.

Spinal neurolysis

Subhash Jain

Introduction 228
Anatomy relevant to spinal neurolysis 229
    Anatomy 229
    Historical perspective 231
Hyperbaric spinal neurolysis 232
    Unilateral intrathecal neurolysis 232
    Bilateral intrathecal neurolysis 232
Hypobaric spinal neurolysis 234
Conclusion 237
    Key learning points 237
Further reading 238

Introduction

In spite of advances in cancer diagnosis, treatments, and an increased survival rate, the undertreatment of cancer pain remains a major problem throughout the world. Cancer pain may have various presentations. Careful assessment, understanding painful conditions in cancer, accurate diagnosis for causes of pain, appropriate use of drugs, interventional, psychological, and other available strategies are all essential for improving the well-being of the patient. This chapter will focus on the role of neuroablative treatment for management of intractable cancer pain.

Perineural injections of local anaesthetics have been used therapeutically since the late 19th century following the development of hollow needles by Rynd 1845 and Wood 1855, and the introduction of cocaine by Karl Koller (1884). The application of neurolytics to provide relief of intractable pain has been practised since these techniques were popularized by Dogliotti, Maher, and others. The clinical use of subarachnoid neurolysis using alcohol was reported by Dogliotti using 0.2–0.8mL of absolute alcohol. In 1931, Dogliotti performed his first application of intrathecal injection of alcohol to relieve intractable pain for patients who were too sick to have surgery or had a very short life expectancy. Following his initial paper other physicians reported their experiences for using intrathecal alcohol. The use of intrathecal phenol was reported by Maher in 1957; he also used this extradurally and subdurally. In 1959 Kelley and Nathan injected 10% phenol subarachnoid. In 1963 Maher reported slightly better results using chlorocresol. In the last three decades Racz and Jain injected phenol via a Racz catheter to produce epidural neurolysis. Nathan *et al.* reported non-selective destruction of fibres. However, neither the methods of block nor the neurolytic agents have changed much over the intervening years. Recognition of total pain and integration of neural blockade techniques into a multidisciplinary strategy was an important step forward.

There are various methods for intrathecal neurolysis. A hypobaric technique is used when a solution of lower specific gravity than CSF is injected, e.g. alcohol. Conversely when a hyperbaric chemical, e.g. phenol in glycerine, is used intrathecally the injectate lies in the dependent region. However, infarction due to damage to the nutrient vessels of the spinal cord, followed by persistent neurological injury, is a risk after neurolysis near the cord.

Anatomy relevant to spinal neurolysis

Anatomy

Spinal neural ablative procedures involve injection of a neural destructive agent into CSF to produce pain relief. The spinal cord extends from the medulla oblongata to the lower border of the lumbar 1st or upper border of the lumbar 2nd vertebra (Figure 18.1). Knowledge of dermatomes is critical to safe application of spinal neurolysis (Figure 18.2). The subarachnoid space extends to the lower border of S1 and often to the upper border of S3. Spinal neurolysis can be achieved by administrating a neurolytic agent into the subarachnoid, extradural, or subdural space. A low concentration of 2% chlorocresol or 3–5% of phenol in water will be destructive to C fibres only when injected into the extradural or subdural space. A higher concentration of the agent will affect motor fibres as well as other myelinated sensory fibres; this destructive action can produce patchy and unpredictable effects. The effect of 40% alcohol is equivalent to 3% phenol when it is applied to the rat sciatic nerve. A large number of studies were performed using intrathecal phenol that produces protein denaturation. Phenol has very strong affinities to vascular tissue and this is responsible for its interfering with tissue blood flow. Most of its action is due to its impact on neural tissue by producing neurolysis.

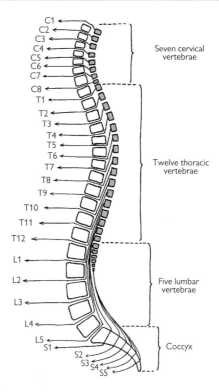

Figure 18.1 Relationship between the origin of spinal nerves from the spinal cord and point of exit from spinal column. Image courtesy of Dr SG Tordoff FRCA FFPMRCA.

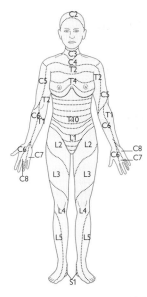

Figure 18.2 Dermatome chart. Image courtesy of Dr SG Tordoff FRCA FFPMRCA.

Historical perspective

In the past five decades the most commonly used agents in the US are 5% phenol in water, phenol in glycerine, 2% chlorocresol in glycerine, or absolute alcohol. The role of phenol and chlorocresol in glycerine is as a hyperbaric solution when injected in the CSF. The use of these agents is for a very limited range of indications, e.g. to treat cancer pain, to relieve spasticity, or to treat severe neuralgia, i.e. base of skull involvement of trigeminal or glossopharyngeal nerves. Chlorocresol produces more motor block compared to phenol; it exerts its effect for up to 24 hours. In contrast to chlorocresol, phenol exerts its effect rapidly due to its rapid absorption.

Hyperbaric spinal neurolysis

When a hyperbaric technique is used for treating intractable pain, careful technique is required to identify the dermatomal levels of pain (Figure 18.2). Once the anatomical location is identified topographically the dermatomal nerve distribution of pain must be documented. Prior to the procedure careful consent is needed that includes risks, benefits, and possible immediate or long-term adverse effects. Any pre-existing neurological deficit must be documented.

Unilateral intrathecal neurolysis

Unilateral intrathecal block is performed with the painful site located in the lateral position and dependent. The dermatomal region is marked with a pen and the body of vertebra is identified. The affected site is aseptically prepared. The goal of the hyperbaric technique is to bathe most of the dorsal root fibres. The needle is placed under X-ray control in the designated space and once the tip of the needle has entered the subarachnoid space the free flow of CSF should be observed (Figure 18.3). The needle is slowly pulled back until the flow of CSF is just present. Once that is achieved 5% phenol in glycerine is slowly injected with the patient lying with the painful part in a dependent and posterior position. The table position is very important to manipulate the flow of phenol, e.g. if the painful site is at L2–L3 and the patient feels paraesthesia in the sacral distribution after injection then the table needs to be put head down so that the neurolytic does not travel to the sacral fibres. During the procedure communication with the patient is very important. The usual doses for various anatomical regions is: thoracic 0.5–1mL and for lumbosacral 0.5–0.6mL. This block can be repeated if pain relief is not adequate. A minimum period of 7–10 days is an ideal waiting time. The block can fail due to tumour infiltration in the subarachnoid space or if the cord is involved in tumour. Meningeal or epidural space infiltration also has a direct effect on the spread of phenol. The most common untoward effects of this procedure include headache, back pain, vascular infarction, spinal cord injury, neurotoxicity, arterial thrombosis, bladder or bowel or sexual dysfunction, paresis, paraesthesia and motor block. A patient with pre-existing neural weakness will be more prone to feel motor weakness.

Bilateral intrathecal neurolysis

Intrathecal bilateral neural block is a strategy for midline pain, e.g. carcinoma of the rectum, pelvis, cervix, or uterus when a patient develops perineal pain. These patients may have already lost bowel, bladder, or sexual function with severe perineal pain. Midline placement of the needle at L4–L5 or L5–S1 level is used and intrathecal phenol in glycerine is slowly injected.

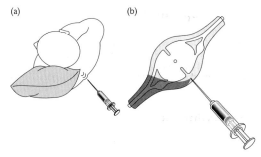

Figure 18.3 Patient position for hyperbaric spinal neurolysis. Image courtesy of Dr SG Tordoff FRCA FFPMRCA.

Hypobaric spinal neurolysis

The most common agent available is absolute alcohol. After subarachnoid injection analgesia is for a shorter period from a few days to a 6-week period. In the early papers a higher incidence of bladder and bowel function disturbances was reported. The fast conducting A and non-myelinated C fibres are damaged when they come in contact with alcohol. During post mortem some patients who have received subarachnoid alcohol showed alcohol affecting the posterior roots as well as degeneration of the posterior column of the cord. Alcohol has a dual action. The initial injection acts like a local anaesthetic; this is followed by destructive and non-selective action on other fibres. The destructive effect depends on concentration, volume, and the area of the spinal root and cord exposed to alcohol.

Patient selection and consent is important. As for an intrathecal phenol the dermatomal distribution of pain and the needle placement site is marked. The major difference between the injection of alcohol versus phenol and glycerine is the position of the patient. As alcohol is a hypobaric solution the painful site is kept upwards in the lateral position (Figure 18.4). Alcohol has a specific gravity of 0.807 when injected in CSF and the CSF specific gravity is 1.007–1.008. The patient should be kept in static position and the goal is to get the alcohol into the dorsal root. The recommended initial dose is 0.8–1.5mL; it must be slowly administered.

As well as the lateral position, the procedure can be done in prone position with a pillow under the abdomen and following the injection of alcohol bilateral analgesia can be produced with this technique. In this position the goal is to bathe both sides of the dorsal roots. This is best achieved by using hypobaric alcohol; the table should be tilted head down so the hypobaric alcohol will be able to float in the desired dermatomal level. The amount of alcohol should be restricted to 1.5–2mL maximum in one treatment and it should be injected in increments of 0.2mL to localize its spread. Patients usually report burning sensation in the dermatome covered by injected alcohol and this helps in further adjustments of table tilt to allow spread of alcohol in desired dermatome. The patient should be observed for any motor blocks, or severe burning/paraesthesia. The patient must be kept in the same posture for 30–45 minutes so the injected alcohol is fully bound to the desired dorsal roots. Following the procedure there is an immediate analgesic effect followed by continuous neurolysis for 72 hours.

The indications and contraindications for alcohol and phenol neurolysis are listed in Boxes 18.1–18.4 and include causes for inadequate pain relief and various complications.

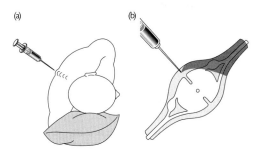

(a) (b)

Figure 18.4 Patient position for hypobaric spinal neurolysis. Image courtesy of Dr SG Tordoff FRCA FFPMRCA.

Box 18.1 Indications for spinal neurolysis

- History of advanced malignancy
- Life expectancy of <6 months
- Preferred patient with compromised bowel and bladder function
- Poor candidate for surgical options or neurosurgical interventions
- Poor physical condition
- Failed treatment or severe side effects from analgesics
- To improve quality of life.

Box 18.2 Contraindication for subarachnoid neurolysis

- Patient refusal
- Spinal cord tumour
- Tumour of the spinal column in the needle entry region
- Diffuse widespread distribution of pain
- Pain not due to tumour.

Box 18.3 Causes of inadequate relief from subarachnoid neurolysis

- Inadequate neurolytic agent
- History of local tumour involvement, i.e. epidural carcinomatosis
- Radiation therapy-related changes or cancerous infiltration in spinal pathways
- Disease progression.

Box 18.4 **Complications of subarachnoid neurolysis**
- Painful reaction to neurolytic due to depositing it in wrong area
- Post-dural puncture headache
- Infection
- Impairment of sensory function
- Bladder and bowel incontinence; sexual dysfunction
- Meningism
- Transverse myelitis
- Paraplegia, paresis
- Arachnoiditis
- Cauda equina syndrome
- Chronic dysaesthesia
- Vascular infarction.

Conclusion

Spinal neurolysis has been in use for almost 100 years. Various chemicals, e.g. alcohol, phenol, ammonium salts, and glycerol, are used to produce subarachnoid neurolysis. During the last three decades this technique has been used less due to improvements in drugs and percutaneous neurolytic techniques. In spite of this there is still a role for these blocks in carefully selected patients to manage intractable pain.

Key learning points

- In spite of advances in management of intractable pain, the neurolytic procedures still play a vital role in managing severe cancer pain.
- These are simple, cheap, and well known for managing complex and difficult cancer pain.

Further reading

Hollis PH, Malis LI, Zapulla Ra (1984). Neurological deterioration after lumbar puncture below complete spinal subarachnoid block. *J Neurosurg*, **64**(2), 253–6.

Lifshitz S, Debacker LJ, Buchsbaum HJ (1976). Subarachnoid phenol block for pain relief in gynecologic malignancy. *Obstet Gynecol*, **48**(3), 316–20.

Stovner J, Endressen R (1972). Intrathecal phenol for cancer pain. *Acta Anaesthesiol Scand*, **16**(1), 17–21.

Swerdlow M (1982). Medicolegal aspects of complications following pain relieving blocks. *Pain*, **13**(4), 321–31.

Swerdlow M (1989). Intrathecal and extradural block in pain relief. In Swerdlow M, Charlton JE (eds) *Relief of Intractable Pain*, 4th edn, pp. 223–57. Amsterdam: Elsevier.

Trigeminal interventions for head and neck cancer pain

Devjit Srivastava and Manohar Sharma

Introduction 240
Relevant anatomy 241
  Applied anatomy for interventions 241
Patient assessment 242
Management options 243
  Foramen ovale-based interventions 243
  RF/balloon microcompression of trigeminal ganglion 243
  RF thermocoagulation of the Gasserian ganglion 243
  Balloon microcompression of the Gasserian ganglion 243
  Contraindications 243
  Technical aspects of RF thermocoagulation of Gasserian
    ganglion 243
  Technical pearls 244
  Technical aspects trigeminal balloon microcompression 245
  Technical pearls 247
  Aftercare post RF or balloon compression 247
  Complications of RF of Gasserian ganglion/balloon
    microcompression 247
  Peripheral procedures 247
Conclusion 248
  Key learning points 248
Further reading 249

Introduction

Head and neck cancer usually refers to malignant tumours that arise in the mucosa of the oral cavity, pharynx, larynx, nasal cavity, and paranasal sinuses. Pain is a significant problem with head and neck cancers. Everdingen *et al.* reported an overall pain prevalence of >50% in patients with all cancer types; the highest cancer subtype was head and neck cancer, with a pain prevalence of 70%.

Pain may be caused by the cancer itself. Pain can also be caused by cancer invading nerve, muscle, mucosal damage, and tumour pressure. Treatments for cancer like surgery, radiotherapy, and chemotherapy by themselves can also cause pain. One of the commonest manifestations is mucositis-related pain. At times, the pain may be unrelated to cancer and may be myofascial or related to temporomandibular joint dysfunction.

Trigeminal neuralgia may occur in head and neck cancer patients as a result of trigeminal nerve involvement either due to cancer or its therapy. This form of trigeminal neuralgia is termed secondary or tumour-related trigeminal neuralgia. If there is accompanying numbness related to trigeminal nerve involvement in association with constant pain, then the diagnosis is trigeminal neuropathy and in this case the neuroablative interventions are contraindicated. In this chapter we discuss the role of trigeminal interventional procedures in providing relief from pain in trigeminal distribution.

Relevant anatomy

The trigeminal nerve is a mixed nerve that consists primarily of sensory neurons. It exits the brain on the lateral surface of the pons, entering the trigeminal ganglion within a few millimetres. The trigeminal ganglion corresponds to the dorsal root ganglion of a spinal nerve. Three major branches emerge from the trigeminal ganglion. Each branch innervates a different dermatome (Figure 19.1). Each branch exits the cranium through a different foramen (Figure 19.2):

- The 1st division, V1, ophthalmic nerve, exits the cranium through the superior orbital fissure, entering the orbit to innervate the globe and skin in the area above the eye and forehead.
- The 2nd division, V2, maxillary nerve, exits through the foramen rotundum, into a space posterior to the orbit, the pterygopalatine fossa. It supplies middle third of face.
- The 3rd division, V3, mandibular nerve, exits the cranium through an oval hole, the foramen ovale. It supplies lower third of face.

Applied anatomy for interventions

- For foramen ovale-based interventions, if the needle trajectory is too posterior, it may enter foramen lacerum through which carotid artery passes.
- If the needle trajectory is too anterior, needle may enter orbital cavity leading on to retro-bulbar haemorrhage.
- If the needle is too medial and deep, injury to cavernous sinus and cranial nerve supply to eyeball is possible.

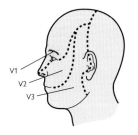

Figure 19.1 Diagram showing part of face supplied by various divisions of trigeminal nerve. Image courtesy of Dr SG Tordoff FRCA FFPMRCA.

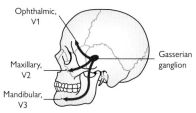

Figure 19.2 Anatomy of trigeminal nerve. Image courtesy of Dr SG Tordoff FRCA FFPMRCA.

Patient assessment

According to the British Pain Society cancer pain guidelines detailed pain history, examination, and investigations should be performed. Additional history of comorbidities and carer/family history along with other relevant medical history must be taken.

The history should include key features of oncology history. One should find out the type of tumour, duration since diagnosis, treatments (radiotherapy, chemotherapy, or surgery) which the patient has undergone.

Trigeminal neuralgia in head and neck cancer is diagnosed if the patient has
- Paroxysmal attacks of pain lasting from seconds to 2 minutes in the area subserved by the trigeminal nerve.
- Pain should have one of the following characteristics:
  - Sharp, shooting, stabbing
  - Precipitated from trigger areas.
- No pain in between attacks and absence of background pain. MRI/MRA should be performed to rule out neurovascular conflict and possible role of microvascular decompression.

Management options

For patients with trigeminal area pain, trigeminal percutaneous interventions are usually offered when the pharmacological management of cancer pain (as covered in Chapter 2) has failed.

Additionally, medical treatment for trigeminal neuralgia i.e carbamazepine, pregabalin and gabapentin may be tried initially. If medications are ineffective, invasive procedures as delineated here may be helpful. It is important to discuss the benefits and risks of these invasive procedures.

Foramen ovale-based interventions

- RF, balloon compression, and glycerol injection are well recognized techniques for pain control. Technique for glycerol injection will not be covered in this chapter.
- Apart from technical aspects, consent is very important as patients need to know that it is a neuroablative technique and there is a high chance of numbness, unpleasant dysesthesia, and temporary jaw weakness.

RF/balloon microcompression of trigeminal ganglion

A discussion with the patient regarding expected common risks and benefits of this procedure needs to be undertaken.

RF thermocoagulation of the Gasserian ganglion

- This needs the patient's cooperation with sensory stimulation and retesting after the RF lesion.
- It is not preferred for 1st division trigeminal (ophthalmic) neuralgia.

Balloon microcompression of the Gasserian ganglion

- Preferred for 1st division trigeminal (ophthalmic) neuralgia or pain in ophthalmic distribution.
- The patient and/or operator's preference to have the whole procedure under general anaesthesia.

Contraindications

- Local or systemic infection
- Bleeding diathesis or anticoagulation.
- Numbness in painful area (trigeminal neuropathy).

Technical aspects of RF thermocoagulation of Gasserian ganglion

Preparation

- Consent includes discussion of likely success rate and potential complications. All patients must be warned about the risk of numbness and potential jaw weakness.
- Prepare the patient as for general anaesthesia.
- Position the patient supine on a radiolucent table with a thin pillow under the head.
- High-quality X-ray images are needed (Figure 19.3) as identification of foramen ovale is essential.
- Equipment needed: RF lesion generator, 22G 100mm RF needle with 5mm active tip, thermocouple probe for sensory stimulation and RF lesioning, local anaesthetic, and simple equipment for sensory examination after the heat lesion.

- Strict asepsis is essential. It is usual to administer one dose of prophylactic antibiotic according to the local guidance.
- An anaesthetist must be present to monitor the patient and administer general anaesthesia.

Technique

- The C arm should be positioned with around a 45° caudal tilt and a 15–30° ipsilateral oblique tilt to identify the foramen ovale (Figure 19.3). Minor adjustments may be needed to clearly define its margins.
- Usually the foramen is visualized just medial to condyle of mandible (Figure 19.3). For beginners, it may be beneficial to have experienced colleagues in theatre or an experienced radiologist/radiographer.
- The needle entry point lies just laterally to the angle of mouth (2–3cm). The skin and subcutaneous tissues over this point are infiltrated with local anaesthetic.
- An RF needle is advanced carefully towards foramen ovale (Figure 19.4).
- If targeting the 2nd or 3rd division then enter at about 2cm away from angle of the mouth aiming for the middle third of foramen ovale. If aiming for the 1st division, start about 3cm away from angle of the mouth aiming to medial third of foramen ovale.
- Usually it is possible to have tactile sensation while passing through foramen ovale. This can be very painful and general anaesthesia may be needed at this stage.
- Perform motor stimulation at 2Hz. If there are masseter movements at low sensory thresholds (<0.5V), then advance the needle by couple of mm and retest, until these movements disappear. Check the needle position with a lateral X-ray view.
- Stop general anaesthetic now, wake the patient and perform sensory stimulation at 50Hz. Try to produce paraesthesiae in the affected division of the trigeminal nerve at low thresholds (0.05–0.2V). CSF may drip through the needle; this is entirely acceptable.
- If paraesthesia occurs in the correct division of the trigeminal nerve, then create an RF lesion at 65°C for 60 seconds.
- The patient will need to be anaesthetized for this lesion as it is very painful. After the lesion, check sensory testing in the affected area of face to see whether the patient has developed numbness. If not, the RF lesion will need to be repeated at 70°C and even up to 75°C, until there is objective evidence of numbness.

Technical pearls

- After the RF needle has been inserted through the foramen ovale, check the depth of needle insertion with a lateral view. The needle should not be inserted beyond the clival line as this can be very dangerous.
- Try to avoid inserting the RF needle through the buccal mucosa, as it can introduce infection. Prevent this by inserting one finger into the mouth when initially inserting the RF needle.
- Biplanar imaging facilities help with advancement of needle and checking in two planes at the same time.
- This procedure needs close cooperation between the operator and anaesthetist as the patient may need multiple sleep–awake cycles to produce numbness in the affected division of trigeminal nerve.

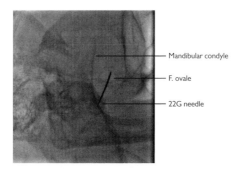

Figure 19.3 Showing 22G RF cannula through foramen ovale in the oblique view. Note the location of foramen ovale medial to the mandible. Reproduced from Simpson *et al.*, Oxford Specialist Handbooks in Pain Medicine, *Spinal Interventions in Pain Management*, Figure 13.4a, p. 244, Oxford University Press, Oxford, UK, Copyright © 2012, by permission of Oxford University Press.

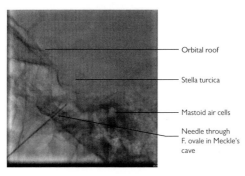

Figure 19.4 Lateral view showing final position of RF needle. Note that the needle stops short of the clival line. Reproduced from Simpson *et al.*, Oxford Specialist Handbooks in Pain Medicine, *Spinal Interventions in Pain Management*, Figure 13.4b, p. 244, Oxford University Press, Oxford, UK, Copyright © 2012, by permission of Oxford University Press.

Technical aspects of trigeminal balloon microcompression

- This may be preferable in patients who cannot tolerate RF lesioning of the Gasserian ganglion. Consent, preparation, position, and image guidance to visualize the foramen ovale is as for the RF technique.
- Equipment: 14G cannula, 4FG Fogarty embolectomy catheter and Omnipaque™ 300 contrast.

- The procedure is carried out under general anaesthesia as the patient's cooperation is not needed.
- A 14G needle is passed under X-ray guidance up to the level of foramen ovale (Figure 19.5). The needle does not go as deep as in the RF technique (Figure 19.4).
- A 4FG Fogarty embolectomy catheter is introduced through the 14G needle. The balloon is inflated with 0.6–0.8 ml of Omnipaque™ 300 for 1 minute, then deflated for 1 minute; two more cycles of inflation/deflation are repeated.
- A pear shape of inflated balloon reflects effective compression of Gasserian ganglion (Figure 19.5). It is reassuring to see medial projection of the inflated balloon on an AP view (Figure 19.6).

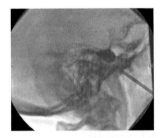

Figure 19.5 Balloon compression: showing pear shape of inflated balloon in Meckel's cave. Reproduced from Simpson *et al.*, Oxford Specialist Handbooks in Pain Medicine, *Spinal Interventions in Pain Management*, Figure 13.6a, p. 246, Oxford University Press, Oxford, UK, Copyright © 2012, by permission of Oxford University Press.

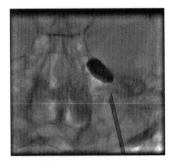

Figure 19.6 AP view showing medial trajectory of inflated balloon. Reproduced from Simpson *et al.*, Oxford Specialist Handbooks in Pain Medicine, *Spinal Interventions in Pain Management*, Figure 13.6b, p. 246, Oxford University Press, Oxford, UK, Copyright © 2012, by permission of Oxford University Press.

- At the end of procedure the needle and Fogarty balloon are withdrawn together. Trying to remove the balloon through the needle may result in shearing of bits of balloon and these may be left behind.

Technical pearls
- The Fogarty balloon should be de-aired to facilitate effective compression of the trigeminal ganglion.
- The 14G needle should be introduced only up to the level of the foramen ovale and no further.
- Transient bradycardia or even asystole may be observed with balloon inflation or inserting the needle through the foramen.

Aftercare post RF or balloon compression
- The patient needs the usual postoperative care and can usually be discharged the next day.
- With careful planning, it can be performed as day case as well. They may need simple analgesics for postoperative pain.
- It is good practice to do a neurological examination the day after and document numbness, jaw weakness, and the presence or absence of a corneal reflex.

Complications of RF of Gasserian ganglion/balloon microcompression
- Temporary jaw weakness (more common with balloon microcompression)
- Cheek haematoma (settles quickly)
- Unpleasant dysaesthesia
- Anaesthesia dolorosa (1–4%, more common with RF)
- Cranial nerves palsy (temporary)
- Very rare complications
  - Corneal ulceration
  - Retro-bulbar haemorrhage
  - Carotid artery puncture
  - Intracranial haemorrhage
  - Meningitis.

Peripheral procedures
- When head and neck cancer patients have pain restricted to the territory of the terminal branches of the trigeminal nerve, then it may be useful to perform a peripheral nerve block with neurolytic agents like absolute alcohol or 6–10% aqueous phenol.
- A trial of local anaesthetic block to test efficacy is recommended before injecting neurolytic agents. These blocks can be targeted to mandibular, maxillary, infraorbital, inframental, supraorbital, and supratrochlear nerve.
- There is a high chance of neuritis and pain relief usually lasts for weeks, rather than months.

Conclusion

- Pain from head and neck cancer can be very disabling to patients and may become a quality of life issue.
- When pain medications do not work, one should consider trigeminal interventional procedures.
- A holistic biopsychosocial assessment of the patient is mandatory.
- For trigeminal distribution pain in V2/V3 territory, RF thermocoagulation of the trigeminal nerve is preferred, whereas balloon compression is preferred for the 1st division.

Key learning points

- For head and neck cancer-related pain specific trigeminal interventions are very effective in medically refractory pain.
- Patient consent is very important for neuroablative techniques as often patients will have long-lasting numbness in the face.
- Better imaging facilities help to localize foramen ovale and hence minimize complications related to inadvertent cannulation of other foramina.
- These techniques should be planned in close collaboration with palliative care or oncologists who may be managing the patient for palliation of cancer.

Further reading

British Pain Society Cancer Pain Guidelines. Available at: ℘ <http://www.britishpainsociety.org/book_cancer_pain.pdf> (accessed 20 April 2013).

Datta S, Pai UT (2006). Interventional approaches to management of pain of oral cancer. *Oral Maxillofac Surg Clin North Am*, **18**(4), 627–41.

Mullan S, Lichtor T (1983). Percutaneous microcompression of the trigeminal ganglion for trigeminal neuralgia. *J Neurosurg*, **59**(6), 1007–12.

Skirving D J, Dan NG (2001). A 20-year review of percutaneous balloon compression of the trigeminal ganglion. *J Neurosurg*, **94**(6), 913–17.

Tatli M, Sindou M (2008). Anatomoradiological landmarks for accuracy of radiofrequency thermorhizotomy in the treatment of trigeminal neuralgia. *Neurosurgery*, **63**(1, Suppl 1),129–37.

Van den Beuken-van Everdingen MH, de Rijke JM, Kessels AG, Schouten HC, van Kleef M, Patijn J (2007). Prevalence of pain in patients with cancer: a systematic review of the past 40 years. *Ann Oncol*, **18**, 1437–49.

Neurosurgical techniques for cancer pain

Paul Eldridge

Treatment of the cause *252*
  Introduction *252*
  Goals of primary surgical procedures for cancer *252*
  Examples for role of surgery *252*
Neuromodulation *254*
  Spinal cord stimulation *254*
  TENS *254*
  Deep brain stimulation *254*
  Motor cortex and transcranial magnetic stimulation *254*
  Intrathecal drug delivery systems *255*
Lesions *256*
  Historical perspective *256*
  Lesioning techniques *256*
  Stereotactic techniques *257*
  Pituitary *257*
  Limbic lesioning for pain—the anterior cingulotomy *258*
  Thalamotomy *258*
  Brainstem lesions for intractable pain *258*
  DREZ lesion and the nucleus caudalis DREZ lesion *259*
  Cordotomy *259*
  Commissural or midline myelotomy *259*
Conclusion *260*
  Key learning points *260*
Further reading *261*

Treatment of the cause

Introduction
The neurosurgical principles of treating pain apply in cancer pain as much as they do in any other situation and these are in the following order:
- Treat the cause
- Neuromodulation
- Neuroablation.

Treating the cause is of necessity at the site of the tumour itself; neuro-modulation techniques, and lesions are performed on the pain pathways, and these can be either spinal or cranial.

It is not practical here to cover this topic other than in principle as one of the goals of the treatment of any cancer is pain relief, and frequently pain—characterized by its novelty to the patient and its relentlessly progressive nature is a cardinal symptom of cancer.

Goals of primary surgical procedures for cancer

Provide a diagnosis
Often the diagnosis may have been made before surgery, but, at times, it may be after surgery.

Cytoreductive
Potentially to cure in its own right, or to facilitate adjunctive treatments such as chemotherapy and radiotherapy, or if cure is not possible then to prolong the disease-free, or progression-free interval, and survival. This is conventionally presented as a Kaplan–Meier type statistic and there is progressively more weight attached to measures such as the disease-free interval as opposed to a simple survival curve. Quality of life measures such as performance status or Karnofsky scores are used, and the partition for measurement purposes of outcome is often set as the ability of the patient to live independently.

Restoration and preservation of function
It is one of the expectations of the surgery for cancer.

Pain relief
It is expected that removal or reduction in size of tumour will help control the pain.

Examples for role of surgery
The earlier listed goals are well illustrated by two neurosurgical examples.

In the case of malignant glioma a presenting feature is frequently pro-gressive headache. Surgical treatment by obtaining tissue establishes the diagnosis; cytoreduction has been shown to be associated with prolonged survival. The more complete the resection the greater the length of sur-vival. Self-evidently the resection, by preventing immediate progression, will preserve existing function; in addition, in that some function is compro-mised by compression of nervous tissue, and tumour inflammation, surgery will often be followed by restoration of function. Finally it is by far and away the best and most immediate treatment for the headache resulting from mass effect.

The second example has been referred to earlier and is the treatment of spinal metastases. It is worth noting that in 90% of cases of metastatic spinal cord compression the first symptom is pain, and the overall outcome is best when this is the only symptom. The publication of a randomized trial comparing surgical management with best medical management of metastatic disease of the spine has altered practice in favour of surgical intervention (chemoradiation is a usual adjunct).

The two groups were decompressive surgery and radiotherapy compared to radiotherapy alone; the trial was stopped early by its data monitoring committee because clear evidence in favour of surgery was established. The significant findings were that more patients in the surgery group were able to walk (84% vs 57% after treatment; those walking retained this ability for a longer time period (122 vs 13 days), the survival time was greater in the surgical group and the need for corticosteroids (daily dexamethasone equivalent dose 1.6mg vs 4.2mg) and opioids (daily morphine equivalent dose 0.4mg vs 4.8mg) was reduced in the surgical group. This is powerful evidence, class 1 evidence, in favour of surgical treatment with all of the goals mentioned previously being achieved. This result was obtained with quite strict, and perhaps too restrictive, selection criteria, so that the recruitment period was quite prolonged despite the trial being stopped early. An issue for this and indeed any trial is to what extent the results can be extrapolated to other patients who might have been excluded from the study by reason of the exclusion criteria of the trial. In fact the statistical levels of significance in this trial were quite robust, suggesting that cases should exist outside the trial criteria that could have benefitted; however, the dangers of extrapolation are obvious and do not need emphasis!

Finally a health economic analysis also suggested that in addition this approach was cost-effective.

Neuromodulation

Spinal cord stimulation

Electrical stimulation is not regularly performed for cancer pain.

The biggest use of electrical stimulation for pain is spinal cord stimulation in which the dorsal columns of the spinal cord are stimulated, paraesthesiae produced, and pain relief obtained. The exact mechanism is still hotly debated; the original philosophy was to interfere with the 'gate' proposed originally by Melzack and Wall, and some form of modulation of the sensory input to the ascending pain pathway still seems likely. Classically nociceptive pain does not respond, and the analgesic effect of stimulation is not reversed by naloxone; in practice, trials are rarely done and it has not been thought appropriate to implant expensive hardware into patients with limited life expectancy. This is perhaps odd as the first use of spinal cord stimulation in 1967 by Shealey was for this indication. This has led to some re-evaluation of the technique, and although no randomized trials exist there are a number of case series (in addition to the original report) in which good pain relief is reported. The other circumstance in which spinal cord stimulation has been employed successfully is to treat postsurgical complications of cancer treatment, such as neuropathic pain due to surgical wounds. However, this is not really included in the concept of cancer pain treatment as the aetiology is not the cancer directly.

TENS

Transcutaneous nerve stimulation is a non-invasive method which has been used in cancer pain. However, from randomized trials evidence as to its effectiveness is equivocal so it does not find widespread use. There is some evidence that it may on occasion be helpful for bone pain. Anecdotally it may be a successful treatment.

Deep brain stimulation

Historically there has been more motivation to pursue deep brain targets, though most of the work has been lesional (neuroablation), and there are no controlled trials, merely observational case series. For nociceptive pain the target used has tended to be the periaqueductal grey, and for neuropathic pain the sensory thalamus. In a review of several series, 23 cases with cancer pain were identified; of these 19 obtained early relief, and 15 long-term relief. There is of course the usual potential for publication bias in this assembly of evidence from case series.

Motor cortex and transcranial magnetic stimulation

In theory, transcranial magnetic stimulation and motor cortex stimulation may find application for cancer pain, though hitherto the techniques have been restricted to non-malignant pains. There is interest in transcranial magnetic stimulation to treat disorders such as depression, and to enhance functional recovery after brain injury. These areas may, therefore, find an application in cancer pain, as in a holistic view of cancer pain these influences are significant i.e. both the direct influences on pain pathways, and those which influence its psychological interpretation by the brain.

Much though not all of this work was carried out some years ago, and before techniques of deep brain stimulation became technologically much more improved. This has been largely due to the increase in the use of deep brain stimulation for movement disorders. There has been a similar improvement in the technology available for spinal cord stimulation, and further techniques of dorsal root ganglion stimulation. These changes and others may lead to a resurgence of the use of deep brain stimulation, spinal cord stimulation, and other types of electrical stimulation for the treatment of the pain of cancer.

Intrathecal drug delivery systems

This topic is covered elsewhere in this book (see Chapter 17). Attention is therefore simply drawn here to a randomized trial of this mode of therapy. Patients with cancer pain were randomized to conventional medical management (CMM), or to have an ITDD system. 84.5% of patients with a drug delivery system had satisfactory pain control compared to 71% without; the ITDD system patients achieved a greater fall in the VAS score, and had less drug toxicity, including less fatigue. All of these effects were statistically significant, but in addition those with a delivery system had improved survival, with 54% alive at 6 months compared with 37% of the CMM group; this last parameter did not quite reach statistical significance ($P = 0.06$). This would imply that these systems are not used as readily as perhaps they should be; however, they do require intense management of the patient, so a physician might consider a lesional technique more practical because of easier aftercare.

Lesions

Historical perspective

Historically, lesions were used more frequently as the systemic techniques for medical management in palliative care were much less refined than they are now. Many will remember the improvements brought about in palliative care by the influence amongst others of Dame Cicely Saunders. Secondly, cancers presented at a much more advanced stage. Thirdly, there are many more modern treatments available for the primary tumour and finally the technologies available for drug delivery, or for electrical stimulation, were so poor that lesional techniques were to be preferred. A clear and remaining advantage of lesional techniques over neuromodulatory methods is that once the lesion is performed then the patient is free of the physician and the hospital, whereas stimulators or drug delivery systems require intense management, the latter particularly so, and this means the patient is more closely dependent on the healthcare system. If independence is viewed as one measure of quality of life then this is clearly a disadvantage.

For this reason there may be a resurgence in the next few years of lesional techniques, and there are emerging technologies, that may make non-invasive lesions practical. It's germane to remember that Lars Leksell originally devised the gamma knife to treat cancer pain (finding that LINAC (linear particle accelerator) technology of that time was insufficiently energetic). His first ideas regarding stereotactic radiosurgery were as long ago as 1951, with the advent of the first 'gamma knife' in 1967.

Lesioning techniques

There are a number of methods for creating lesions. Transection by scalpel or knife is obvious and found in surgical cordotomy. Chemical can be injected such as alcohol; however, other techniques include RF lesioning in which heat is generated electrically at the point of an electrode, using high-frequency stimulus. This is perhaps the most commonly used technique. In this system it is necessary to locate the tip of the electrode accurately in the designated target, and the size and configuration of the electrode defines the shape of the lesion and its precision. Typical lesioning temperatures are around 70–80°C for a time of around 15–45 seconds, and in the brain will create a roughly spherical lesion perhaps 2–3mm in diameter. Similar technology is used for percutaneous cordotomy, and the dorsal root entry zone (DREZ) lesion and the technique is widely used for non-cancerous pain. With this technique it is possible and therefore a frequent practice to perform a test lesion using a much lower temperature, perhaps 40°C, which is reversible. Assessment of efficacy and side effects can be made. In addition, once the electrode is at target, physiological stimulation to activate the neural structures can confirm the physiological location of the electrode in an awake patient.

Another method of causing a lesion is stereotactic radiation using the gamma knife or LINAC-based systems. High-energy photons are produced and aimed precisely at a target. Finally there is interest in percutaneous ultrasound methods. These can create thermal lesions, can be MR guided, and there is the ability to perform test lesioning.

Stereotactic techniques

This term has been used throughout this chapter. It refers to a technique for locating accurately in space a target within the human body, and placing an electrode, biopsy instrument, or lesion generator. Historically it referred to the brain, with a frame attached to the skull with a series of pins; the frame carried fiducials and imaging would be performed that would show the fiducials, and a defined landmark or landmarks in the brain. Once this was done an aim apparatus was attached to the frame in place of the fiducials and the procedure typically allowed an accuracy of 1–2mm to be achieved. Modern computing power has meant that the preferred imaging technique is MRI fused to CT; frameless technology can now be used, and that instead of individual slices being used calculations are carried out using a whole volume. This means that instead of at most 10–20 data points being used, whole datasets of 30–60Mb are routinely used, and sometimes even more than this. Although the systems have been used mainly in the brain, and occasionally the high cervical spinal cord, solutions are now available for most other areas in the body, and these can even function in real time taking account of the patients respiration.

The lesions that have been used follow the pain pathway and can be classified in a similar manner (Table 20.1).

Pituitary

A historical technique dating from the days in which hypophysectomy was practised as an hormonal manipulation in the treatment of certain

Table 20.1 Examples of lesion location

Lesion location	Example
Peripheral nerve	Phenol nerve block
Spinal cord	Anterolateral cordotomy
	DREZ
	Commissural myelotomy
	Nucleus caudalis
Brainstem	Mesencephalotomy
Basal ganglia	Thalamotomy
Limbic circuits	Cingulotomy
Other	Pituitary

cancers, notably breast and prostate, when it was noted that pain relief was a welcome side effect and often immediate. There were a number of different techniques used including open surgery, transsphenoidal surgery, and destructive techniques to the pituitary itself such as RF lesioning, stereotactic radiosurgery, and the placement of yttrium seeds. One of the commoner techniques, promoted by Morrica was the injection of alcohol. Morrica's own results were spectacularly good, but never replicated by others. He claimed >90% pain relief, but a more usual figure was that obtained by Lipton of around 40% with a further 30% obtaining partial relief. There were serious complications as well—which included a mortality, hypothalamic damage, visual damage, and diabetes insipidus. Finally the pain relief was not particularly long-lasting. In Lipton's series only 20% obtained pain relief >3 months. It is not therefore surprising that the method was abandoned when better techniques of primary tumour control came about, and better routes of administration of opioids.

Limbic lesioning for pain—the anterior cingulotomy

Again a historical procedure, though one that might become resurgent. The technique perhaps therefore provides some insight into the neural networks involved in the patient's perception of pain. Recently the cingulate gyrus has become a target for deep brain stimulation; not just for chronic pain but also depression and addiction. In the case of pain the patients appear to no longer find their sensory experience unpleasant. Lesions here therefore hover on the border of psychosurgery; the original motivation to look at this concept came from the notorious practice of leucotomy practised by Freeman. Bilateral cingulotomy is the only procedure that has been associated with improvements in pain. Reported results for cancer pain are all in case series. Typical results are that perhaps two-thirds of patients experience pain relief, but that the effect is time limited with recurrence after only a few months—perhaps as few as three. Better results may be obtained when anxiety and depression accompany the pain.

Thalamotomy

Sensory thalamotomy (ventral posteromedial nucleus/ventral posterolateral nucleus) has been used successfully for the treatment of cancer pain. The indication is widespread pain, or head and neck pain. It is perhaps less efficacious then mesencephalotomy, but has less side effects. It is considered that medial thalamotomy is best for cancer patients with 30–50% gaining pain relief though this is often relatively short-lived. The technique can be done by RF lesioning or using the gamma knife. However, with the former technique patient feedback can be obtained and thus correct localization is aided by patient feedback that is not possible with the radiosurgical method.

Brainstem lesions for intractable pain

Mesencephalotomy can be viewed as a supraspinal form of cordotomy. It is done stereotactically, and the results for cancer pain report 'long term relief that is until death'. Pain relief in up to 90% of patients, though in some series the pain relief rate is very poor at <10%. There are frequent side effects, and in particular oculomotor dysfunction, the lesion being at the level of the superior colliculi.

DREZ lesion and the nucleus caudalis DREZ lesion

The point at which the dorsal roots of a peripheral nerve enter the spinal cord, or in the case of the nucleus caudalis DREZ procedure the bottom part of the adjoining brainstem (the DREZ) is lesioned either physically by cutting or by RF. It is a substantial operation and rarely performed particularly for cancer pain as the recovery time is not trivial. There are a number of small case series only. These report that approximately two-thirds might gain significant benefit.

Cordotomy

Cordotomy, the percutaneous form is covered elsewhere (see Chapter 16); occasionally there is a need to perform open surgical cordotomy. In this unit the indications are bilateral pain (one side is done percutaneously, the other open); technical failure of cordotomy, and metastatic disease within the cervical spinal canal. It may be more effective than the percutaneous technique for pain in the sacral region, though is of greater morbidity being an open procedure.

Despite this, the procedure is of less morbidity than is generally appreciated, and the effects are, in the short term, dramatic. A thoracic laminectomy is performed at least four segments above the spinal level of the pain (some have argued that the procedure should always be at a high thoracic level (T1–T2)), and the dura opened to expose the cord. The anterolateral part of the cord is exposed by rotating the cord (conveniently done using the ligamentum denticulatum), and a lesion made with a small knife. The results are as for open cordotomy and about 50% of patients are satisfied with pain relief at 12 months. There is a risk of development of post-lesioning dysaesthesia, so the technique is solely reserved for pain of malignant origin.

Commissural or midline myelotomy

This is a variant of cordotomy—the principle is that the pain fibres which decussate across the spinal cord are divided. This decussation happens across about four segments in the cord. It has been used instead of a bilateral cordotomy. It has never been performed extensively. A variant was discovered in that a midline lesion at C1 produced analgesia over a wide area, and that limited myelotomy at T10 provided visceral pain relief. Although there is no proven substrate for this procedure, the hypothesis is that within the dorsal column in the midline lies a visceral pain pathway, and this is the substrate of the lesion which does not in postmortem samples even reach the commissure in all cases.

Conclusion

There are a number of procedures available within the neurosurgical armamentarium for the control of cancer pain. Whilst in the main cancer pain
is successfully controlled by medical means, the neurosurgical methods and
in particular the lesional techniques should not be abandoned and probably
have a greater place than has been appreciated; the ability to achieve significant pain relief, without large doses of opioids may well result in improved
quality of life and by itself improved survival.

Key learning points

- There are a number of procedures available within the neurosurgical
  armamentarium for the control of cancer pain.
- The lesional techniques should not be abandoned and probably have
  a greater place than has been appreciated because of the ability to
  achieve significant pain relief, without large doses of opioids.
- Better pain relief without excessive reliance on opioids may well result
  in improved quality of life and by itself improved survival.
- Close collaboration with neurosurgical units specializing in pain control
  can help otherwise very difficult to control cancer pain.

Further reading

Bittar RG, Kar-Purkayastha I, Owen SL, Bear RE, Green A, Wang S, et al. (2005). Deep brain stimulation for pain relief: a meta-analysis. *J Clin Neurosci*, **12**(5), 515–19.

Cetas JS, Raslan A, Burchiel KJ (2011). Evidence base for destructive procedures. In Winn HR (ed) *Youmans Neurological Surgery*, 6th edn, pp. 1835–44. Philadelphia, PA: Elsevier.

Freeman WJ, Watts JW (1948). Psychosurgery for pain. *South Med J*, **41**, 1045–9.

Jones B, Finlay I, Ray A, Simpson B (2003). Is there still a role for open cordotomy in cancer pain management? *J Pain Symptom Manag*, **25**, 179–84.

Leksell L (1951). The stereotaxic method and radiosurgery of the brain. *Acta Chir Scand*, **102**, 312–19.

Lihua P, Su M, Zejun Z, Ke W, Bennett MI (2013). Spinal cord stimulation for cancer-related pain in adults. *Cochrane Database Syst Rev*, **2**, CD009389. doi: 10.1002/14651858.CD009389.pub2

Morrica G (1974). Chemical hypophysectomy for cancer pain. In Bonica JJ (ed) *Advances in Neurology*, Vol. 4, pp. 707–14. New York: Raven Press.

Nauta HJ, Soukup VM, Fabian RH, Lin JT, Grady JJ, Williams CG, et al. (2000). Punctate midline myelotomy for the relief of visceral cancer pain. *J Neurosurg*, **92**(2), 125–30.

Patchell RA, Tibbs PA, Regine WF, Payne R, Saris S, Kryscio RJ, et al. (2005). Direct decompressive surgical resection in the treatment of spinal cord compression caused by metastatic cancer: a randomised trial. *Lancet*, **366**(9486), 643–8.

Raslan AM, Cetas JS, McCartney S, Burchiel KJ (2011). Destructive procedures for control of cancer pain: the case for cordotomy. *J Neurosurg*, **114**(1), 155–70.

Smith TJ, Staats PS, Deer T, Stearns LJ, Rauck RL, Boortz-Marx RL, et al.; Implantable Drug Delivery Systems Study Group (2002). Randomized clinical trial of an implantable drug delivery system compared with comprehensive medical management for refractory cancer pain: impact on pain, drug-related toxicity, and survival. *J Clin Oncol*, **20**(19), 4040–9.

Thomas KC, Nosyk B, Fisher CG, Dvorak M, Patchell RA, Regine WF, et al. (2006). Cost-effectiveness of surgery plus radiotherapy versus radiotherapy alone for metastatic epidural spinal cord compression. *Int J Radiat Oncol Biol Phys*, **66**(4), 1212–18.

Yen CP, Kung SS, Su YF, Lin WC, Howng SL, Kwan AL (2005). Stereotactic bilateral anterior cingulotomy for intractable pain. *J Clin Neurosci*, **12**(8), 886–90.

Peripheral nerve blocks including neurolytic blocks

Andrew Jones

Rationale for peripheral nerve blocks 264
   Introduction 264
   Rationale 264
   Pain service and nerve blocks in hospice settings 264
Common nerve blocks 265
   Intercostal nerve block 265
   Periosteal pecking 265
   Suprascapular nerve block 265
   Intercostobrachial nerve block 265
   Femoral nerve block 266
   Trigger point injection 266
Neurolytic techniques 267
Conclusion 268
   Key learning points 268
Further reading 269

Rationale for peripheral nerve blocks

Introduction

Peripheral nerve blocks with local anaesthetic with or without steroid may give analgesia that lasts for longer than the duration of action of the local anaesthetic in some patients, i.e. several weeks or even months. One patient, in my experience, had 8 months of pain relief. This may be due to the temporary loss of nociception causing longer-lasting changes in the nervous system that generate chronic pain.

Rationale

Patients with cancer may suffer from pain due to neuralgia in a nerve distribution that may not be directly due to the cancer. However, they are also often distressed from their diagnosis and they may have a very limited prognosis. A successful nerve block may give considerable relief in these patients. However, incident pain due to metastases or pathological fracture is unlikely to be relieved by nerve block; in this situation the patient should be carefully assessed and referred for surgery or radiotherapy or if unsuitable for either of these, then for spinal infusions or neuroablative techniques.

Chronic pain seen in the general pain clinic may arise in patients with cancer unconnected to the malignant process. Again, the coexisting diagnosis of cancer implies a more interventional approach than that used in the pain clinic.

In my practice, nerve block is considered (although not always indicated or performed) in any case of pain refractory to conventional palliation. If the pain relief is only for the duration of action of the local anaesthetic, a continuous catheter technique should be considered. All interventions should only be performed with the informed consent of the patient after a discussion of risks and benefits.

Pain service and nerve blocks in hospice settings

Patients being treated in a hospice may not be well enough for transfer to hospital or may be distressed by leaving, even for a few hours, the comforting environment engendered by hospice care. Consequently, the interventional pain service should be considered as a bedside service wherever possible. The same standards of care including asepsis, intravenous access where indicated, and resuscitation still apply. The issue of resuscitation from adverse effects of nerve block such as intravascular injection need to be carefully discussed with a patient who has a current 'Do Not Actively Resuscitate' order. The patient's relatives and carers should ideally be involved in these discussions if that is the patient's wish. There is more scope with outpatient attendees for referral for more specialist techniques.

Analysis of a year's interventional activity in one hospice showed that the commonest interventions in descending order were trigger point injections, intercostal nerve blocks, suprascapular nerve block, and femoral nerve block.

Common nerve blocks

Intercostal nerve block

Chest wall pain may be associated with tumours (primary or secondary) of the lung, surgery, or may arise spontaneously (intercostal neuralgia). Mesothelioma is an increasingly common cause. On examination it is usually associated with a tender rib or ribs. Intercostal nerve blocks often give several weeks or months of pain control. The patient should be warned that the pain may increase during the injection. The patient should be carefully counselled about the risk of pneumothorax, as the benefits of pain control will be negated by the need for a chest drain. In addition patients with lung cancer frequently have coexisting chronic obstructive pulmonary disease. Pneumothorax may make shortness of breath more distressing and may even precipitate respiratory failure.

The intercostal block should be performed at the site of maximum rib tenderness. The needle is passed under the rib to enter the neurovascular bundle in the intercostal groove. My practice is to inject 5mL 0.5% bupivacaine with steroid if not contraindicated. An ultrasound-guided technique (if available) may help to reduce risk and improve efficacy; this applies to most other techniques in this chapter.

Periosteal pecking

Intercostal neuralgia may be relieved with periosteal pecking; as this technique involves hitting the rib rather than accessing the neurovascular bundle the risk of pneumothorax is much reduced. An acupuncture needle is used to tap rapidly on the tender rib. Many patients get pain relief after a minute or two of pecking. A month or more of relief may be expected and the occasional patient will have long-term analgesia. If pain control is not satisfactory with periosteal pecking, intercostal nerve block may be indicated.

Suprascapular nerve block

Shoulder pain may arise spontaneously or be secondary to pre-existing osteoarthritis. It may develop in response to disuse of a painful arm, for example, the pain that follows breast surgery. While referral to a shoulder surgeon should be considered, rapid relief may be obtained on the spot with a suprascapular nerve block. The nerve block may be the main treatment or a temporary measure whilst definitive treatment is awaited. If the suprascapular notch is avoided, there is no risk of pneumothorax. The nerve is blocked by inserting the needle on to the bony surface of the lateral supraspinous groove; 7–8ml 0.5% bupivacaine with or without steroid is injected.

Intercostobrachial nerve block

Chronic pain is common after surgery for breast cancer. It may include arm and hand pain. A number of patients with such pain will be tender in the axilla. They may benefit from an intercostobrachial nerve block. In practice, the injection should be placed in the point of maximum tenderness. Complications are avoided by keeping the injection superficial, thus avoiding intravascular injection or brachial plexus block; 4–5ml 0.5% bupivacaine with or without steroid is injected. Chronic pain after breast surgery may be associated with shoulder pain. A suprascapular nerve block will provide analgesia to allow access to the axilla by abducting the arm.

Femoral nerve block

Femoral nerve block may give pain control in femoral neuralgia, hip/knee pain, and pain arising from the femur. Femoral neuralgia may arise spontaneously, be a consequence of hip or pelvic surgery, or be associated with femoral lymphadenopathy. Hip and knee pain is often due to coexisting osteoarthritis. If the pain has suddenly increased a pathological fracture should be excluded. If present, this should be treated with surgical fixation, if possible. If surgery is contraindicated, a continuous infusion of local anaesthetic via an indwelling catheter is more likely to give pain control than a single-shot technique.

The patient should be warned of the possibility of motor block with consequent risk of falls. It may be advisable to provide crutches. The femoral nerve is identified using a nerve stimulator. Ultrasound may be useful but is unlikely to be affordable by many hospices. My practice is to inject 15ml 0.125% bupivacaine with or without steroid. The low concentration of local anaesthetic reduces the incidence of motor block. Other pain specialists advocate a higher concentration and accept motor block as a consequence. If there is poor pain control, then cordotomy should be considered as it can be very effective and does not produce motor block.

Trigger point injection

While trigger point injection is not a nerve block it is included here for two reasons. Prolonged pain relief from a trigger point injection probably comes from the same neuromodulatory effects as nerve block. More importantly, pain and disability from trigger points is common and easily treated. Examination of the patient with refractory pain should include a thorough hunt for trigger points. Pain caused by trigger points may radiate in a non-dermatomal pattern. Consequently, a large area of pain may be controlled by a trigger point injection. As the complications (bruising and infection) are rare and the increase in pain during the injection transient, very few patients are unsuitable for such injection. Trigger points are identified by eliciting pain on palpation. Injection of 0.5% bupivacaine with or without steroid may give weeks or months of pain control. Failure to get control may be due to missing or unmasking of further trigger points. Re-examination will reveal this. Trigger point injections may be repeated as often as the patient can tolerate it.

Neurolytic techniques

Neurolytic techniques are avoided in my practice due to the incidence (10%) of neuritis that may result in worse pain than treated. Pain that has no, or short-lived, control using single-shot techniques can be managed using catheter techniques with continuous infusion. If the peripheral nerve is unsuitable for a catheter, central neural blockade (epidural or intrathecal) should be considered as described in other chapters in this book. If the pain is exclusively unilateral, then anterolateral cordotomy may be appropriate.

Conclusion

The palliative care patient with pain refractory to conventional medication or suffering from medication toxicity should be carefully assessed. If the pain is in the territory of a peripheral nerve or associated with trigger points, then intervention using local anaesthetic with or without steroid may give weeks or months of pain control.

Key learning points

- Palliative care patients may achieve significant and long-lasting pain control from simple one-shot techniques.
- Peripheral neurolytic techniques provide short-term benefit only with the risk of neuritis and deafferentation pain.

Further reading

Bandolier. *Chronic Pain After Surgery*. Available at: ℛ <http://www.medicine.ox.ac.uk/bandolier/band103/b103-4.html> (accessed 20 April 2013).

British Pain Society (2010). *Cancer Pain Management*. Available at: ℛ <http://www.britishpainsociety.org/book_cancer_pain.pdf> (accessed 20 April 2013).

Section C

Collaboration between services

22 Role of collaboration between pain medicine
   and palliative medicine   273
23 Control of complex pain at the end of life
   in hospice or community setting   285

Role of collaboration between pain medicine and palliative care

Heino Hugel

Background and current status of collaboration 274
  Introduction 274
Liverpool model of collaboration between pain and palliative
  medicine 275
  Benefits of collaboration for palliative care physicians 275
  Benefits of collaboration for pain physicians 276
  Logistics: assessment and procedures locations 276
Case discussion 277
  Learning points from case discussion 277
Practical aspects of service delivery 279
Other benefits of collaboration between pain and palliative
  medicine 281
Conclusion 282
  Key learning points 282
Further reading 283

Background and current status of collaboration

Introduction

The need for access to interventional pain medicine in cancer pain management is well described in the literature. Different studies have shown that 70–90% of cancer pain can be managed following the WHO ladder. However, for the remaining 10–30% advanced pain management techniques including invasive procedures may be required. A number of national cancer policies such as the cancer manual or the Supportive and Palliative Care Guidance from NICE in the UK stipulate that interventional pain medicine should be an integral part of standard cancer care. In addition the *Mesothelioma Framework* highlights that patients with this condition should have access to percutaneous cordotomy. However, access to interventional pain management for cancer pain at least in the UK is patchy and joint working between palliative medicine and pain physicians is not that well established.

- Multidisciplinary working in a team of healthcare professionals from different professional backgrounds is an established way of working in palliative as well as pain medicine. However, collaboration between clinical specialties is variable.
- A survey by Linklater *et al.* from 2002 of palliative medicine physicians in the UK showed that only 53% held joint consultations with pain specialists. In addition 80% of consultations were held with the pain service only when required. Only 15% of surveyed physicians had access to regular pain specialist sessions. Also, only 40% of participants felt that regular anaesthetic input was essential, suggesting a lack of awareness of the need for invasive pain management.
- Another paper by Kay *et al.* from 2007 reciprocated this survey with pain physicians in the UK. This showed that 54% of the surveyed pain physicians received five referrals or fewer for cancer pain per year. Only a quarter stated that they held joint consultations with palliative care doctors. There was also significant variation in what procedures different pain services were able to offer for management of cancer pain, with only very few centres providing more complex procedures such as percutaneous cordotomy or other nerve destructive interventions.
- On the positive note, this paper showed that pain physicians who had regular allocated clinic time for cancer pain patients were receiving more patient referrals and performed more procedures.

Liverpool model of collaboration between pain and palliative medicine

The author of this chapter is the palliative care link of a joint pain/palliative care clinic at a large university hospital complex in the North West of England. We hold a weekly clinic where patients are seen usually within a week of referral.

There is full access to a wide range of procedures and access to other specialities such as neurosurgeons and oncologists as required.

The clinic was founded in the 1990s and now sees referrals from a supraregional catchment area.

From our experience there are clear benefits from collaboration between pain and palliative care specialists. If patients are seen jointly, they meet both specialists at the same time. This avoids duplication of consultation and gives the patients immediate access to the required full information about conservative and invasive pain management options.

For more complex procedures it is also beneficial to have more than one consultation to assure assessment at different time points and fully informed consent. By working closely with referrers a regular joint clinic fosters a culture of patients being referred at earlier stages in their disease when they are well enough to benefit from invasive procedures.

Collaborations takes some time to develop and build up, but this time is well invested and should be an essential part of a joint clinic. It is only possible to build these relationships if clinicians have adequate allocated time to do the clinic.

Our clinic started quite informally and initially dealt with local referrals. Since holding a formal clinic and working with actual and potential referrers our referrals have increased and we have almost half our referrals from out of our region. Another benefit from collaboration is learning from each other, i.e. for the clinicians involved.

Benefits of collaboration for palliative care physicians

- Palliative care physicians should first of all recognize that access to invasive pain management is important for their patients. Since they are usually hosting these patients for holistic symptom management they should also aim to host the joint consultations with pain specialists.
- It is important for palliative care physicians to be aware of the range of procedures that are available locally and for which procedures, e.g. percutaneous cordotomy, they need to refer to larger pain management centre.
- Referrals should be specific and not simply state referral for a nerve block as this may raise unrealistic expectations for patients. It is better to state that a referral is being made for an opinion otherwise patients can become frustrated and angry, or may demand inappropriate procedures.
- Palliative care physicians should also see invasive procedures as part of comprehensive cancer pain management that has in many cases a place alongside conservative management options.

- Invasive procedures should not be seen as a last resort when all else has failed. This often leads to late referrals and denies the patient an appropriate procedure due to reduced general performance status.

Benefits of collaboration for pain physicians

- Pain physicians on the other hand should differentiate cancer pain from more chronic pain-related management techniques.
- Timely assessment and ready access to required procedures is key for patients with limited life expectancy like cancer patients. This requires flexibility and availability in assessment and providing a selected procedure.
- Pain physicians should also take into account the patient's other symptoms and treatment preferences and put the pain problem into context of other clinical and environmental issues.
- Choosing the right procedure is also important. Patients at the end of life are often frail overall, and may well only tolerate one procedure. It is therefore important to choose the procedure that is most likely to benefit the pain problem in one session and last for the duration of the illness with as few side effects as possible.
- Neurolytic procedures in particular are helpful in this regard from our experience.
- These were more frequently employed in the past, before better conservative management options were developed. However, they have been, perhaps unfairly, criticized as side effect prone and causing unpleasant neuralgic syndromes post procedure.

Logistics: assessment and procedures locations

- To guarantee successful procedures and minimize complications, it is important to provide the appropriate environment for pre- and postprocedure care and for the procedure itself.
- The specialist palliative care environment, i.e. hospice or specialist palliative care unit, is ideally suited to host the patients for pre- and postprocedure care. There patients benefit from holistic management of pain as well as other symptoms.
- Also, as patients with complex pain problems are often on high doses of opioids, the safe down-titration of these is best done in a specialist palliative care environment rather than general medical wards.
- However, patients equally benefit from having the procedures in the appropriate environment, i.e. operating theatre. This guarantees that procedures are done in optimal conditions, aseptically, and with access to appropriate imaging if required.
- Only in cases where patients are clearly not well enough and if there is a suitable procedure that can be done outside the theatre environment should procedures be done wherever the patient is located.

Case discussion

The following case illustrates the benefits of joint working. An 88-year-old retired man was referred to the joint pain/palliative care clinic from a local hospital 80 miles away. There he had presented 2 weeks prior to referral following a suicide attempt with an overdose of morphine due to severe uncontrolled incident pain from a recurrent chondrosarcoma in his left hip. He had been treated with nail fixation and radiotherapy in the past. Over the preceding 2 months pain in his left hip had steadily escalated. He was virtually pain free at rest in bed, but simple movement or nursing procedures would cause excruciating pain in his left hip and down his left leg. This was managed with escalating doses of morphine up to 500mg/24 hours, paracetamol 1g four times a day, gabapentin 600mg three times a day, diclofenac 50mg three times a day, and Sevredol® as required. In addition he required Entonox® for any nursing intervention. He was on a general hospital ward and his declared biggest wish was to die at home. There was in addition a difficult family situation with children living far away from home and difficulties in managing the care. So here was a combination of a severe pain problem, psychological support needs following suicide attempt, as well as care and family issues.

Following telephone consultations between the referrer and the pain and palliative care physicians, the patient was transferred to our hospital palliative care unit. On arrival the patient was opioid toxic with myoclonic jerks and pinpoint pupils. The patient agreed to a percutaneous cordotomy and so in advance of this, the morphine was gradually reduced to 200mg/24 hours within a 3-day period without deterioration of pain control and some improvement in levels of toxicity. The patient also received psychological support and the family were brought up to date with clinical developments and care was planned for discharge. The patient then underwent the cordotomy at the pain centre which resulted in marked improvement in pain control. Following the procedure the morphine was further down-titrated in the specialist palliative care environment to 100mg/24 hours. The patient was able to be nursed pain free following the cordotomy with no need for Entonox®. The palliative care team then arranged transfer back to a local hospice where he stayed for a week before being discharged home where he died 4 weeks later.

Learning points from case discussion

- Complex pain problem with incident pain, i.e. pain on movement which is difficult to control with conservative management.
- Pain itself is not life threatening, but due to required treatments such as analgesia can lead to life-threatening complications such as toxicity from medication and infections.
- Complex analgesic regimen with added toxicity is best managed in specialist palliative care environment.
- Pain in these patients is rarely an isolated problem. Pain needs to be seen in context with other symptoms and ongoing issues. This patient had psychological needs such as dealing with his terminal illness, his recent suicide attempt, and his complex care situation which all needed to be addressed alongside the pain problem.

- The patient was referred late. Incident pain pattern should have alerted clinicians to refer the patient sooner for an invasive procedure before crisis developed.

Locally achievable pain management options like epidural catheter were not feasible in this case due to lack of community support. One could argue that all specialist palliative care units should aim to have access to invasive pain management for more commonly needed procedures like neuraxial infusions.

Practical aspects of service delivery

Due to the volume of patients requiring procedures in our area, particularly percutaneous cordotomy, we sometimes have to admit patients to the general hospital. We tend to restrict this to the patients who are overall better in their performance status and not on high doses of opioids. We have had cases where either opioids were reduced by ward staff too quickly or doses were omitted and then patients have had opioid withdrawal, and we have also had patients who were given their original opioid dose on admission on discharge when, due to successful procedures, the opioid dose had been significantly reduced. This then resulted in the patient being significantly toxic at home. In response to this we have developed a care pathway particularly for percutaneous cordotomy which we are now implementing in the general hospital and the hospice. This covers all important care issues including review of opioid doses.

In our clinic around 50% of the patients referred will eventually undergo an invasive procedure. The reasons for not undergoing a procedure include too far advanced disease and not being deemed fit enough to undergo a procedure. Some pains may not be suitable for an intervention. But sometimes also the patients opt not to have a procedure even if there would be an indication for a procedure. We always aim to give a balanced view on benefits and risks of procedures. Sometimes our consultations are mainly about exploring further management options in case the conservative route is not successful enough. Just knowing that something else could be done if needed is often sufficient for patients to carry on with their conservative management. We also see it as our role to support referrers with conservative management options and signposting. Within our catchment area specialist palliative care and pain services are not all developed to the same level, particularly in some rural areas cover can be patchy. We have done consultations sometimes over mobile speaker phone, trying to find a suitable pain management option for referrer and patient.

It is also important to highlight the need for rehabilitation as an important part of the joint working theme. If cancer pain is severe enough and difficult to control with conservative measures it can become an overriding symptom for patients and reduce both physical as well as psychological function significantly. Once the pain is improved following a successful procedure, a process of rehabilitation is important to improve function. In addition, physiotherapy in particular can help patients to be able to tolerate a procedure. We not infrequently use the physiotherapist to increase patients' ability to lie flat for a cordotomy or to sit upright for insertion of a neuraxial needle or a saddle block.

Equally important is for the nursing staff involved in a patient's care to have a good awareness of the interventional procedures and their side effects. This is relevant to both theatre staff as well as general nurses. Particularly for procedures that are harder to tolerate for patients and where success of procedure is significantly linked to patient cooperation like percutaneous cordotomy, supportive theatre and ward nursing staff are invaluable. Well-trained nursing staff are also particularly important in care of neuraxial infusions. Here good cooperation with community as well as specialist palliative care nursing staff is essential to allow patients with these devices to be cared for at home. There can be problems with care of lines and pump devices in the community. These need to be anticipated and protocols and guidelines need to be developed with the community staff before lines are inserted and infusions titrated in the inpatient setting.

Other benefits of collaboration between pain and palliative medicine

- An important part of the collaboration as highlighted earlier is continuous learning. Through the collaboration itself pain and palliative care physicians can learn from each other. This is important for successful functioning of the clinic as well as further professional development. It is also a very enjoyable part of joint working.
- In addition education of referrers and other involved healthcare professionals is also relevant. Invasive pain management for cancer pain is not equally well developed in all areas and it is hence important to make clinicians aware of the importance of this approach.
- We have been involved in a number of educational initiatives locally, nationally, and internationally and see this as a significant part of our work commitment. The evidence base for quite a few of the invasive procedures is also limited. Most evidence comes from case series. Randomized controlled trials are difficult to conduct as numbers of procedures are often small and placebo control is ethically not an option.
- Evidence is crucial both in terms of clinically justifying invasive procedures as well as for commissioners of services who in times of tight resources will only want to commission procedures with proven efficacy. We conduct continuous prospective audit for quality purposes as well as evidence gathering.
- We have presented our data at national and international conferences and have been involved in a national consensus research project into the use of percutaneous cordotomy for mesothelioma-related pain.
- Collaboration with other centres is important to increase the number of cases. We have been involved in setting up a national registry for percutaneous cordotomy. This approach exists commonly for a number of specialities and can be useful again for quality control as well as scientific purposes.

Conclusion

Key learning points
- Collaboration between palliative care and pain physicians in management of cancer pain is crucial.
- Joint clinics with dedicated clinical time in job plans should be the preferred model to deliver care.
- Suitable environment for assessment and procedures is important. Procedures ideally to be done in theatre, assessments and pre- and postprocedure care in specialist palliative care setting.
- Close collaboration with referrers is important to build up activity and get referrals at the right time.
- Involvement of clinicians in education and research is important as there is currently not enough awareness and a dearth of quality literature around invasive pain management.

Further reading

Chambers WA (2008). Nerve blocks in palliative care. *Br J Anaesth*, **101**(1), 95–100.

Finnegan C, Saravanakumar K, Sharma M, Nash TP, Corcoran GD, Hugel H (2008). The role of epidural phenol in cancer patients at the end of life. *Palliat Med*, **22**(6), 777–8.

Kay S, Husbands E, Antrobus JH, Munday D (2007). Provision for advanced pain management techniques in adult palliative care: a national survey of anaesthetic pain specialists. *Palliat Med*, **21**(4), 279–84.

Linklater GT, Leng ME, Tiernan EJ, Lee MA, Chambers WA (2002). Pain management services in palliative care: a national survey. *Palliat Med*, **16**(5), 435–9.

Mesothelioma Framework (2007). Available at: ℘ <http://www.mesothelioma.uk.com/editorimages/DOH%20Framework%20for%20Mesothelioma.pdf> (accessed 20 April 2013).

National Cancer Peer Review-National Cancer Action Team (2008). *Manual for Cancer Services 2008*. Available at: ℘ <http://www.healthcare-today.co.uk/doclibrary/documents/pdf/ 351_ Manual_for_cancer_services_2008.pdf> (accessed 6 May 2013).

Valeberg BT, Rustoen T, Bjordal K, Hanestad BR, Paul S, Miaskowski C (2008). Self-reported prevalence, etiology, and characteristics of pain in oncology outpatients. *Eur J Pain*, **12**(5), 582–90.

Zech DF, Grond S, Lynch J, Hertel D, Lehmann KA (1995). Validation of WHO Guidelines for cancer pain relief: a 10-year prospective study. *Pain*, **63**(1), 65–76.

Control of complex pain at the end of life in hospice or community setting

Umesh K. Gidwani and Stephen Berns

Management of complex pain 286
    Introduction 286
    General approach to complex pain 286
    Specific hospice considerations for pain management 286
    The hospice comfort kit 287
Analgesics for patients in hospice 288
    Mild pain analgesics 288
    Moderate pain analgesics 288
    Moderate to severe pain analgesics 289
    Opioid management for the hospice patient 291
    Adjuvants for neuropathic pain 291
    Adjuvants for bone-related cancer pain 292
    Adjuvants for malignant bowel obstruction-associated pain 292
    Other adjuvants for cancer pain 292
Ethical concerns for pain management in the community hospice
    setting 293
    Undertreatment in cancer populations 293
    Common misconceptions regarding opioids 293
    Addiction and abuse worries in opioid therapies 294
    Principle of the double effect 295
Interventional pain management 296
    Soft tissue and joint injections 296
    Vertebroplasty and kyphoplasty 296
    Neural blockade and neurolysis 297
Other non-pharmacological methods for pain relief in
    hospice 299
    Palliative radiation therapy 299
    Radiation therapy for bone metastases 299
    Complementary and alternative therapies for pain 300
Controlled sedation for refractory pain 301
    Prior to initiating sedation 301
    Starting the sedation 302
    Ethical concerns with palliative sedation 302
Conclusion 303
    Key learning points 303
Further reading 304

Management of complex pain

Introduction

Pain is very prevalent and common in the cancer population. It has the potential not only to cause physical distress but also to affect the patient's functional status, psychological and emotional state, and social life, particularly when it is severe. Studies of patients in their last week of life reveal that up to 35% describe pain as severe or intolerable. Fortunately, pain is quite treatable and when following the WHO framework on pain relief, up to 90% of individuals with cancer are effectively treated.

General approach to complex pain

The most important step to assuring adequate pain control in the community hospice setting is an accurate assessment of pain. Failure to properly assess pain is often the most common cause of poor pain control:

- Pain scales can be helpful tools in systematically approaching the patient's pain and reassessing interventions.
- Asking about subjective descriptions of pain can help diagnose aetiology and guide treatment plans to accomplish pain relief.
- It is important to take the individual patient's experience into account and to apply methods of treatment to the individual. The right dose of an analgesic will vary from person to person and the correct dose is the one that relieves the patient's pain without causing unmanageable side effects.

As we learned earlier in this book, using the WHO's cancer pain relief guidelines can help to achieve pain relief and these can be summarized in five phrases:

- By the mouth
- By the clock
- By the ladder
- For the individual
- Attention to detail.

Specific hospice considerations for pain management

Because most community hospices have limited resources and most patients are homebound and/or bedbound, there are a few considerations that clinicians should think about when choosing a pain regimen:

- Route of intervention—for patients who cannot take oral medications but require opioid pain management, one may consider a transdermal formulation, subcutaneous, or oral solution.
- Cost—due to higher cost, some advanced pain treatments such as interventional techniques and radiotherapy may not be offered at all hospices.
- Burden of treatment—some treatments require more interventions, more monitoring, or having the patient leave their home to receive the intervention. These burdens may outweigh the potential benefits of the treatment.

The hospice comfort kit

The comfort kit—also known as the emergency kit, e-kit, or hospice kit—is a prescribed set of medications that are kept in a patient's home to be used in the event of an emergency. It enables the family or hospice team to treat any distressing symptoms as quickly as possible. A telephone number to reach the hospice provider on call should also be readily at hand.

The actual contents of the kit vary depending on the hospice agency and the hospice diagnosis. Most contain medications for pain, anxiety, nausea, insomnia, and breathing problems. Examples of medications in a hospice comfort kit and the symptoms they treat are as follows:

- Morphine liquid—pain and dyspnoea
- Lorazepam—anxiety, nausea, or insomnia
- Atropine drops—oropharyngeal secretions ('death rattle')
- Haloperidol tablets—agitation and terminal restlessness
- Prochlorperazine tablets or rectal suppository—nausea and vomiting
- Bisacodyl rectal suppository—constipation
- Phosphate enema—refractory constipation
- Other medications may be included depending on the hospice diagnosis. For example, a patient with a brain tumour who is at risk for seizures may have diazepam suppositories included in their comfort kit.

Analgesics for patients in hospice

Mild pain analgesics

Paracetamol and NSAIDs are the usual first steps in treatment of cancer pain in the hospice community setting.

Paracetamol

- Paracetamol has analgesic and antipyretic activities.
- At low dose it has minimal toxicity but at higher doses it can cause fatal liver and kidney damage.
- Paracetamol is best used for mild nociceptive pain and in patients with persistent fevers.
- Can be useful in suppository form when patients no longer have the ability to take oral medications.

> *Doses:* 325mg, 500mg, 650mg (oral); 120mg/5mL, 250mg/5mL, or 500mg/5mL (solution)
>
> *Frequency:* every 4–6 hours
>
> *Formulations:* tablets, capsules, solution, rectal, injection (IV)
>
> *Maximum dose:* 4g/day; 3g/day for elderly; 2g/day in liver disease.

NSAIDs

NSAIDs have both analgesic and anti-inflammatory components.

- Vary in effectiveness but commonly cause adverse GI and renal side effects. Additionally, chronic NSAID use has been associated with increased risk of cardiovascular disease.
- NSAIDs are useful for patients in mild pain with an inflammatory component, such as bone pain (see Table 23.1).

Table 23.1 NSAID formulations and doses

Ibuprofen	Oral	200–400mg (2.4g max)
Naproxen	Oral or rectal	250–500mg
Ketorolac	Injection (IV, IM, SC)	10–30mg (90mg max)
Diclofenac	Oral, transdermal	50mg three times a day (oral), 1.3% patch
Celecoxib	Oral	200mg twice a day

Moderate pain analgesics

Codeine

Codeine is a weaker opioid agonist that is metabolized by the hepatic cytochrome enzyme CYP2D6:

- It is available in both tablet and syrup formulations and can be used for moderate pain and relief of cough.
- Because of its route of metabolism, it has many drug–drug interactions and may not be suitable for patients with renal or liver disease.

Doses: 15mg, 30mg, 60mg (tablet), 10mg/5mL (solution)

Frequency: every 4–6 hours

Maximum dose: 240mg in day

Formulations: tablet and syrup.

Tramadol

Tramadol is a weak opioid agonist that also has noradrenergic and serotonin-reuptake activity:

- Metabolized by both CYP3A4 and CYP2D6.
- It has many opioid-like side effects such as nausea, vomiting, dizziness, and drowsiness. Hallucinations can occur and it has the potential to lower the seizure threshold.
- Can have serious drug–drug interactions that may lead to adverse effects such as serotonin syndrome.
- Available in both an immediate- and extended-release (ER) form.

Doses: 50mg (IR), 50–400mg (ER)

Frequency: every 4–6 hours (IR); every 12–24 hours (ER)

Maximum dose: 400mg

Formulations: tablets and capsules.

Moderate to severe pain analgesics

Morphine

Morphine is a strong mu receptor agonist and is usually the first line of treatment for patients with pain in the community hospice setting.

- Metabolized by the liver, metabolites are eliminated by the kidney. Patients with renal and/or liver disease are at risk for drug toxicity.
- Does not appear to have a clinically relevant ceiling effect to analgesia
- Relative potency varies according to route of administration and individual patient (see dose equivalent tables for details)
- The oral solution form is easy to use in the community setting as it is highly concentrated and can be given in a small 1mL syringe.

Doses: 10mg, 15mg, 20mg, 30mg (IR); 15mg, 20mg, 30mg, 50mg, 60mg, 80mg, 100mg, 200mg (ER); 5mg, 10mg, 20mg, 30mg (rectal); 2mg/mL, 4mg/mL, 20mg/mL (solution)

Frequency: every 3–4 hours (IR); every 8–24 hours (ER)

Formulations: tablets, capsules, solution, and injection (IV, IM, SC) 5mg, 10mg, 20mg, 30mg (rectal); 2mg/mL, 4mg/mL, 20mg/mL (solution).

Oxycodone

Oxycodone is used for moderate to severe pain:

- Alternative opioid for those who develop side effects to morphine.
- Metabolism and elimination are less dependent on the liver and kidneys and more suitable than morphine for patients with renal or liver disease. Caution is still advised.

- Also available in oral solution, which can be helpful in patients who have difficulty with oral intake.

Doses: 5mg, 10mg, 20mg (IR); 5mg, 10mg, 20mg, 40mg, 80mg (ER); 5mg/mL, 10mg/mL (solution)

Frequency: every 3–4 hours (IR); every 12 hours (ER)

Formulations: tablets, capsules, solution.

Hydromorphone

Hydromorphone is a very potent opioid that is often used also as an alternative to morphine.

- Widely used in North America since diamorphine is not available.
- Although its metabolism is similar to morphine, it seems to have less toxicity in patients with renal and liver disease. Caution is still advised.

Doses: 2mg (SR), 4mg (SR), 8mg (SR), 16mg (SR), 24mg (SR) (PO); 3mg (rectal)

Frequency: every 3–4 hours

Formulations: tablets, capsules, injection (IV, IM, SC).

Fentanyl

Fentanyl is a semi-synthetic opioid that is 75–100× more potent than morphine:

- Metabolized in the liver to inactive metabolites, safe to give in patients with renal disease and liver disease.
- Can be applied transdermally; beneficial in those patients who have difficulty taking oral medications.
- Note—the transdermal patch takes about 12 hours to work after first application and does not reach steady state until 48 hours after application. It is therefore not appropriate in patients who need rapid titration of medication for adequate pain control. A fentanyl patch should only be used in those patients with stable opioid requirements.
- Heat can increase the rate of absorption of fentanyl patches and sweating decreases the rate of absorption for fentanyl patches and it is important to counsel and monitor for these conditions.
- Available in oral form which is used for incidental pain, while the patch is used for continuous baseline pain control.
- Side effects are similar to that of morphine but has less potential effect for constipation.

Doses: 12, 25, 50, 75, 100 micrograms/hour (patch); 200, 400, 600, 800, 1200, 1600 micrograms (PO)

Frequency: every 48–72 hours (transdermal); every 20–30 minutes, four doses maximum (PO)

Formulations: transdermal, transmucosal, and injection (IV, IM, SC).

Methadone

Methadone is a synthetic opioid agonist as well as an NMDA (N-methyl-D-aspartate) antagonist. It is generally effective in patients with severe cancer pain but can also be used for neuropathic pain.

- Methadone is metabolized by the liver by the CYP3A3/4 isoenzyme and converted to inactive metabolites. Excreted through faeces, not through the kidneys. Therefore, it is a good choice for patients with liver and renal disease.
- Has a long half-life in plasma of about 24 hours but it can range from 13–100 hours for some individuals. This makes it a difficult drug to titrate.
- Methadone should only be used by those who have experience using it.
- Can interact with many different drugs including phenytoin, phenobarbital, fluconazole, and SSRIs.

Opioid therapy may not be adequate alone in patients with severe pain and

Doses: 5mg (tablet); 1mg/mL, 10mg/mL (solution)

Frequency: every 8–12 hours

Formulations: tablets, solution, injection (IV, IM).

it may be appropriate to give the patient an adjuvant to the opioid regimen depending on the aetiology of the pain.

Opioid management for the hospice patient

Given that most hospice patients have advanced disease and often present with severe pain, opioids are regularly used in the community setting. Opioids are safe and effective, and are appropriate for the management of cancer-related pain. It is critical for the hospice provider prescribing opiate therapy to:

- Systematically approach starting dosing and titrations
- Monitor opiate-related side effects
- Monitor effectiveness of treatment.

There are numerous side effects to these medications (please see Chapter 2). Constipation is almost universal and it is important to start laxatives in patients on opioids and monitor closely for complications of this symptom.

Adjuvants for neuropathic pain

Although opioids are usually not the first line therapy for neuropathic pain, they are often given in conjunction with other medications. The following medications are often used for hospice patients:

- First-line agents: tricyclic antidepressants, gabapentin, pregabalin, duloxetine
- Second-line agents: other antiepileptics, alpha-2 adrenergic agonists (such as tizanidine), cannabinoids, NMDA receptor antagonists (such as ketamine), benzodiazepines (such as clonazepam).

Adjuvants for bone-related cancer pain

Patients with multifocal bone pain usually are managed first with NSAIDs and an opioid:

- Glucocorticoids rather than NSAIDs can be used also on a short-term basis.
- Other medications that have been shown to be advantageous in bone-related pain for hospice patients are bisphosphonates, denosumab, and calcitonin.
- Some of these medications can be quite expensive and it is important to review the risks/benefits prior to starting these medications.

Adjuvants for malignant bowel obstruction-associated pain

Bowel obstruction is a well-recognized complication in patients with advanced intra-abdominal or pelvic tumours and can often lead to intolerable abdominal pain:

- Along with opioids, anticholinergics such as hyoscine which can be applied transdermally, or glycopyrronium bromide which can be injected, can help decrease gut motility and intraluminal secretions.
- A somatostatin analogue such as octreotide can be dosed at 0.1mg twice daily to achieve the same effects.

Other adjuvants for cancer pain

These drugs have been shown to have potential in improving pain management along with opioids for all types of cancer-related pain.

Glucocorticoids

Glucocorticoids can often alleviate symptoms such as pain, nausea, fatigue, anorexia, and improve overall quality of life.

They are very beneficial in patients with pain associated with capsular expansion or ductal obstruction, lymphoedema, and increased intracranial pressure.

- Although the risk of long-term toxicity can include myopathy, immunosuppression, psychotomimetic effects, and hypoadrenalism, often for hospice patients whose life expectancy is limited, the benefits of the treatment outweigh these risks.
- Important to monitor patients for these side effects and titrate the medication should they become problematic.

Alpha-2 adrenergic agonists

Alpha-2 adrenergic agonists (such as tizanidine and clonidine) have been used as general adjuvants for chronic cancer-related pain:

- Can be administered orally, transdermally, and intraspinally.
- Side effects may include somnolence, dry mouth, and hypotension.

Cannabinoids

Cannabinoids may help to treat cancer-related pain in addition to nausea and anorexia:

- Most common side effects for these medications are dizziness, somnolence, and dry mouth.

Topical anaesthetics

Topical anaesthetics such as lidocaine or capsaicin have been used to treat cancer-related pain mostly for focal or regional pain syndromes.

Ethical concerns for pain management in the community hospice setting

Undertreatment in cancer populations

Despite our best efforts, the rate of undertreatment for cancer pain may be over 40%. Moreover, the odds of undertreatment can be twice as high for minority patients. Causes for undertreatment are:

- Clinicians' lack of knowledge and skills.
- Clinicians' reluctance to prescribe drugs due to concern of side effects, legal concerns, or a fear of hastening death.
- Patients may underreport pain for many reasons, including a desire to be liked by clinicians or concern of distracting physicians from aggressive antineoplastic therapies.
- Patients may not take medications because of the fear of addiction or side effects.
- System-wide impediments to optimal analgesia due to financial constraints, limited number of and access to specialists, or incentive structures that do not prioritize pain management.

It is important to remember that uncontrolled pain results in unnecessary suffering, decreased ability to cope with illness, interference with activities of daily living, extended or repeated hospital admissions, disruption of other anticancer therapies, and poor patient and family satisfaction scores.

Awareness of undertreatment and the willingness to confront its causes are key steps toward improving outcomes.

Common misconceptions regarding opioids

It is important for hospice clinicians to know the general misconceptions regarding opioid therapy for pain management so that they can educate and prevent undertreatment or poor adherence.

'Opioid therapy leads to addiction'

- When prescribed appropriately to relieve pain, there is no indication that opioids lead to addiction in acute pain management.
- Studies have demonstrated that the incidence of addiction is <5% for most patients with cancer-related pain.

'Effective opioid therapy can be achieved when used on an "as needed basis"'

- For patients with continuous pain, medications provided around the clock have a much better impact on pain management, quality of life, and have fewer side effects.

'Opioids should not be given at the end of life because of the risk of respiratory depression'

- Opioids rarely lead to respiratory depression if used appropriately.
- Just like in any procedure, treatment with opioids carries its risks—including respiratory depression. Unlike most procedures, this adverse risk, if it does occur, is easily reversed by naloxone. This risk does not outweigh the benefit of giving the drug.

- It is also important to note that respiratory depression does not occur in isolation, but always in the context of oversedation and mental clouding. These precursors to respiratory depression allow for a careful titration and/or reversal of the opioid.

'Opioids hasten death'
- Opioids are unlikely to hasten death if used in an appropriate manner by a skilled clinician.
- In fact, withholding pain medications is not appropriate when it may reduce a patient's suffering.

Addiction and abuse worries in opioid therapies

Opioids are potentially abusable drugs and safe prescribing requires consideration of the risks associated with drug abuse, addiction, and diversion. Because of the public health consequences of opioid abuse, it is important that clinicians assume responsibility for risk management when potentially abusable drugs like opioids are prescribed for legitimate medical purposes.

Identifying individuals who are at greater risk for developing addiction is a first step to risk management because these individuals will likely benefit from co-management of opioid therapy with an addiction specialist. The following simple questions have been used to identify at-risk individuals:
- Is there a personal history of alcohol or drug abuse?
- Is there a family history of alcohol or drug abuse?
- Does the patient have a major psychiatric disorder?

Although most individuals do not develop addiction or drug abuse when being treated for cancer-related pain, it is important to take the necessary steps to monitor and prevent abuse:
- Determine treatment goals with patients, e.g. goals may not be complete pain relief but improved functional status.
- Informed consent—patients should know the risks and benefits for the treatments.
- Treatment agreements—putting the agreement in writing can facilitate communication between the clinician and patient. Having the patient sign the agreement provides documentation of their discussion and empowers the patient.

Agreements have been shown to be effective in improving communication and often include:
- Agreement to obtain prescriptions for a class of controlled medication from only one clinician and, preferably, from one designated pharmacy.
- Agreement to take the medication only as prescribed.
- Acknowledgment that patients are responsible for arranging refills during regular office hours (not on weekends or evenings).
- Agreement that violation of the terms of the agreement may result in discontinuation of the controlled medication.

For those at high risk, one should consider adding the following:
- Prescribing methods—frequent prescriptions with small quantities.
- Testing for drug abuse—periodic urine drug testing to ensure abstinence from non-medical controlled substances such as marijuana.

- Pharmacological choices—because of concern about street value and abuse liability, the decision might be made to offer treatment with an opioid with a lower abuse potential (e.g. methadone or transdermal fentanyl) or no additional short-acting opioid drug for breakthrough or incident pain, again because of the assumption that these agents are relatively more enticing to those predisposed to drug abuse.

Principle of the double effect

Patients and clinicians often have a misperception of the risk of hastening death by treating pain with opioids. They can also be unsure about the borders of aggressive pain management with controlled sedation for intractable symptoms, physician-assisted suicide, and euthanasia. However, failure to treat the pain can increase patient and family suffering.

- The WHO states that patients have a right to have their pain treated.
- In the US, the Supreme Court ruling in *Vacco* v *Quill* (117 S.Ct. 2293 (US 1997)), stated that 'suffering patients have a constitutionally cognizable interest in obtaining relief from the suffering that they may experience in the last days of their lives'.
- The Catholic Church states 'Even if death is thought imminent, the ordinary care owed to a sick person cannot be legitimately interrupted. Painkillers may be used to alleviate the sufferings of the dying, even at the risk of shortening their days'.

Hospice clinicians are therefore faced with the difficulty of balancing these concerns with their duty and moral obligation to treat pain.

The principle of the double effect stipulates that an intervention having foreseen harmful effects inseparable from the beneficial effect is justifiable if the following are true:

- The action is morally good or neutral.
- The intended outcome is important enough to justify the possible bad effect, where efforts are undertaken to minimize risk of the bad effect.
- The agent intends the good effect and not the bad, either as a means to the good effect or as an end itself.

In other words, administering pain medication to relieve pain is morally justified when the relief of the patient's pain is the clear objective and is important enough to justify the possible adverse effect of sedation that may result in the unlikely outcome of death.

Interventional pain management

For the vast majority of patients with cancer-related pain, pharmacological treatment is effective and well tolerated. However, despite optimization of opioid therapy and the use of adjuvants, a minority of patients with cancer pain do not obtain satisfactory relief with first-line analgesic therapy. When adequate pain relief cannot be achieved through pharmacological means, interventional approaches offer an important alternative, a fourth step in the WHO pain ladder.

Interventional therapies consist of a very diverse group, most of which are non-destructive and performed using needles mostly at the bedside. Interventional therapies include injections, for local relief or nerve blocks, for nociceptive pain.

Good candidates for interventional pain management are patients in whom:

- Conventional pharmacological therapies are unsuccessful in achieving pain goals or side effects are intolerable/unacceptable.
- The specific intervention is likely to provide good analgesia, with minimal or acceptable side effects.
- The benefits of pain relief outweigh the surgical risks.

For most hospice patients, the cost of these procedures often outweighs the prolonged benefit of these procedures and may not be suitable interventional risks for patients with limited life expectancy.

It is important, however, for hospice providers to know about these procedures since these patients may have already undergone these procedures and their pain is still being managed by the interventions.

Soft tissue and joint injections

- Injections into soft tissue and joints are the easiest and most common interventions performed although performed less often for cancer-related pain.
- These injections do not necessarily have to be performed by specialists but hospice or general practice clinicians who are comfortable and familiar with the procedures.
- These injections are designed for patients with pain who have a focal area of myofascial pain or joint pain and no contraindication to injection (such as a coagulopathy or infectious risks). If successful, pain can often be relieved for days to weeks.
- An injection of 1–3mL of dilute local anaesthetic such as 0.25% bupivacaine or 1% lidocaine with or without a glucocorticoid can be given directly into the painful site.

Vertebroplasty and kyphoplasty

Vertebroplasty and kyphoplasty have been used to relieve cancer-related pain that originates from vertebral collapse, likely from metastatic neoplastic disease:

- Vertebroplasty involves the percutaneous injection of bone cement under fluoroscopic guidance into a collapsed vertebral body.

- Kyphoplasty involves the introduction of inflatable bone tamps into the vertebral body that restore the height of the vertebral body, creating a cavity that can then be filled with bone cement.
- The risk of adverse outcomes is low under experienced physicians, but serious complications have occurred, including spinal cord compression and paraplegia.
- Often this procedure is reserved for patients who have persistent and severe back pain that is refractory to steroid, bisphosphonate, and opioid therapy.

Neural blockade and neurolysis

Neural blockade consists of any procedure that delivers an agent for the purpose of modulating nociceptive afferent input to the central nervous system. This can apply when either a non-destructive analgesic or a neurolytic drug is injected.

Non-neurolytic analgesic blocks

Non-neurolytic analgesic blocks can be performed using bolus injection or continuous infusion of a local anaesthetic:

- Can be further divided into somatic or sympathetic neural blocks.
- Visceral cancer pain, which can be difficult to control with opioids and adjuvants, is especially suited to sympathetic neural blockade.
- Performed using an infusion of a local anaesthetic, which can be delivered via a catheter that is placed into the epidural space or one whose tip is placed adjacent to a peripheral nerve or nerve plexus.
- The single injection often lasts for short-term duration and often a device is needed to sustain adequate pain control.

Epidural and intrathecal infusions

Epidural and intrathecal infusions are used for patients who need continuous infusion of pain medications that either require high doses of systemic medications or have intolerable side effects:

- An epidural catheter can be tunnelled under the skin and connected to an external pump that delivers the drug continuously.
- Epidural infusions of a local anaesthetic may be combined with opioids and other drugs such as clonidine.
- Epidural delivery permits analgesia to be restricted to fewer dermatomes, but drug doses up to 10-fold higher are needed, possibly producing more systemic side effects
- A catheter can also be placed for intrathecal continuous delivery as well which does not require as high a dose but may have more devastating risks for infections or permanent neurological effects.
- A patient who has pain that is refractory to systemic pharmacotherapy and a life expectancy of days to weeks may benefit from a percutaneously placed catheter with an external pump.
- If survival is likely to be measured in months, the catheter can be tunnelled under the skin to reduce the risk of dislodgement and serious infection.
- Both fixed-rate and programmable pumps are available.
- Implanted catheters and infusion pumps are generally viewed as cost-effective if estimated life expectancy is 3–6 months or more.

Neurolytic techniques

Neurolytic techniques produce pain relief by destroying afferent neural pathways or sympathetic structures that are involved in pain transmission:

- These techniques are mostly reserved for patients with limited life expectancy.
- Neural destruction can be achieved with chemical neurolysis, surgery, cryotherapy, or RF thermal coagulation. Chemical neurolysis with alcohol and phenol are most commonly used in patients with cancer-related pain.

Common sympathetic nerve blocks

Coeliac plexus block

The coeliac plexus is responsible for transmission of nociceptive information for the abdominal contents:

- Most successful in pain management for pancreatic cancer and upper abdominal visceral involvement.
- Complications can include orthostatic hypotension, back pain, diarrhoea, abdominal aortic dissection, and paraplegia.

Superior hypogastric block

The superior hypogastric ganglion transmits nociceptive information from the pelvis. This block is most often used for patients with ovarian and other gynaecological cancers.

Interpleural block

Often used for patients with oesophageal cancer or metastasis to the ribs. It is performed by introduction of an infusion catheter into the pleural space.

Other non-pharmacological methods for pain relief in hospice

Palliative radiation therapy

Radiotherapy is another modality used for pain management in the hospice setting that can work in conjunction with pharmaceutical agents. As opposed to radiotherapy with intent to treat, the goal of palliative radiotherapy is to address distressing symptoms such as pain—most commonly from bone metastases, spinal cord compression, and fungating masses.

Because treatments cannot be given in the home setting, often shorter courses of therapy with higher doses are given to prevent the burden of transporting to the treatments.

Before making decision to do RT, it is important to:
- Assess the balance between anticipated functional/symptomatic benefit versus time spent receiving treatments and acute toxicities.

It is important to note, that most hospices will only pay or arrange for RT if:
- There are symptoms of pain, bleeding, or neurological catastrophe.
- The patient is expected to live long enough to experience benefit (>4 weeks).
- Benefits outweigh logistic burdens.

Radiation therapy for bone metastases

Radiation therapy for bone metastases can be divided into two types delivered by external beam radiation therapy (EBRT) and radiopharmaceuticals.

External beam radiation therapy

EBRT is designed for single or a limited number of bone sites:
- EBRT to a local field can provide pain relief in 80–90% of cases, with complete response in 50–60% of patients.
- EBRT in the US is most commonly delivered as 30Gy in 10 fractions.
- Multiple clinical trials have demonstrated that 8 Gy×1 is as effective as 3–4Gy×5–10 doses.
- Single dose treatment has been associated with higher rates of retreatment and pathological fractures but is often recommended in those patients where the burden of transportation to treatment outweighs the benefits.
- During therapy, some patients may experience a transient worsening of pain in the first few days of radiation therapy, lasting for 2–3 days.

Radiopharmaceuticals

Bone-targeting radioisotopes are most appropriate for patients with multiple painful lesions:
- The most common radioisotopes are strontium-89 and samarium-153 that localize to area of osteoblastic activity.
- Radioisotopes are likely equal in efficacy in pain relief to EBRT and are more beneficial when there are multiple sites.

Malignant spinal cord compression can occur in up to 3% of all cancer patients (most common in multiple myeloma = 8%):
- Pain is the most common symptom (present in 80–95% of cases).
- For hospice patients who are not surgical candidates because of limited survival and goals of care, EBRT can achieve up to 70% of pain relief.
- EBRT therapy can be dosed as 8Gy×1 or 2Gy×20 doses.
- Should be given along with glucocorticoids.

Complementary and alternative therapies for pain

The management of moderate pain in hospice patients may be improved by the adjunctive use of non-invasive psychological and integrative therapies. These strategies may provide pain relief with fewer drug side effects and may improve physical and psychosocial functioning. Data from randomized trials and meta-analysis are imperfect but have demonstrated potential for the utility of:
- Psychosocial interventions of these techniques which may include cognitive behavioural interventions
- Mind–body therapies
- Meditation
- Music therapy
- Biofield therapies
- Massage
- Acupuncture.

Controlled sedation for refractory pain

Pain management from medications, interventions, and complementary therapy can be quite successful with acceptable pain control achieved in 90–95% of patients. However, there is a small group of patients where these methods fail to relieve the patient's suffering leading to intractable distress towards the end of life. Controlled sedation for refractory pain, also known as total, palliative, or terminal sedation can be defined as sedation for intractable distress in the dying:

- The use of sedation has been reported to be anywhere from 2–50% of hospice patients.
- Indications for sedation often include anxiety/psychological distress, dyspnoea, delirium/agitation, and occasionally pain.
- Controlled sedation should only be implemented after the medical situation has been carefully assessed, a thorough discussion with the patient and family has taken place, and, if possible, consent has been obtained with the goals of care clearly established. Patients should meet the following criteria:
  - Aggressive efforts short of sedation fail to provide relief.
  - Additional invasive/non-invasive treatments are incapable of providing relief.
  - Additional therapies are associated with excessive or unacceptable morbidity, or are unlikely to provide relief with a reasonable time frame.
- Of note, respite sedation can also be useful. This is a time limited trial (usually 24–48 hours) of controlled sedation in an attempt to break the cycle of psychological suffering.
- Sedation may be relatively light, or deep; it may be continuous and anticipated to last until death, or temporary.
- If patients have been on opioid therapy for chronic pain this should be continued in addition to the sedation.
- Once the use of sedation has been activated, ongoing information should be provided to family and staff, questions should be answered, and ethical and legal implications should be clarified.
- Once the desired effect is achieved, the sedation is no longer increased.

Prior to initiating sedation

Ensure thorough discussion of proposed treatment plan and expected outcomes with the patient (if able), all family members, and all medical staff (physicians, nurses, therapists, nursing aides, chaplain, etc.):

- Review plans for use of artificial nutrition/hydration—ensure treatment plan has been discussed (either stopping or continuing) and documented with patient/family and medical team.
- Document informed consent discussion and write 'do not attempt resuscitation' order.
- Assure a peaceful, quiet setting, with a minimum of intrusions.
- Confirm patient/family desire for chaplain/spiritual support prior to starting sedation.
- Review medication and treatment orders—discontinue orders not contributing to comfort (e.g. vital sign monitoring, blood glucose checks).

Starting the sedation

Many drugs have been used to provide effective sedation; there are no controlled trials comparing efficacy:

- Sedation may be accomplished with any of a large number of drugs, the most common of which is benzodiazepine, but it can also be accomplished by barbiturates or propofol.
- Opioids are not useful agents for palliative sedation since they provide only transient sedation and may result in side effects including worsening delirium, myoclonus, and respiratory sedation in opioid naïve patients.
  The following list shows starting doses for the use of sedating drugs including the bolus dose and a starting continuous infusion. The intravenous infusion should be titrated to achieve the desired level of sedation:
- Midazolam (SC, IV): 5mg bolus, 1mg/hour
- Lorazepam (SC, IV): 2–5mg bolus, 0.5–1.0mg/hour
- Thiopental (IV): 5–7mg/kg/hour bolus, then 20–80mg/hour
- Pentobarbital (IV): 1–3mg/kg bolus, 1mg/kg/hour
- Phenobarbital (IV, SC): 200mg bolus (can repeat every 15 minutes), then 25mg/hour
- Propofol (IV): 20–50mg bolus (may repeat), 5–10mg/hour.

Ethical concerns with palliative sedation

- Several studies indicate that, when used appropriately, palliative sedation does not hasten the death of palliative care patients overall. Even when matched for adverse prognostic variables, sedated patients did not have an accelerated demise.
- Depending on their underlying condition, patients may survive sedation for days to many weeks. Titration to primary effect is what distinguishes sedation for intractable symptoms from euthanasia and forms the legal, ethical, and moral framework for sedation for intractable symptoms as an alternative to patient-assisted suicide or euthanasia.
- The clear distinction is the intent to relieve pain and suffering.

Conclusion

Key learning points

- Pain is the most common symptom in hospice patients; accurate assessment of pain and prompt and adequate management of pain is paramount.
- Clinicians providing care for these patients should have expert knowledge of the key principles of effective pain management.
- Hospice patients may have a greater need for systematically escalating doses of potent opioids to achieve efficacious pain control.
- For difficult to manage pain as well as pain in special situations, other modalities such as interventional techniques or complementary therapies may be used to achieve better pain control.
- In cases where pain cannot be achieved by treatment with medications or interventions for hospice patients, controlled sedation can be an effective treatment for intractable distress.

Further reading

Bhaskar AK (2012). Interventional management of cancer pain. *Curr Opin Support Palliat Care*, **6**(1), 1–9.

Chow E, Zeng L, Salvo N, Dennis K, Tsao M, Lutz S (2012). Update on the systematic review of palliative radiotherapy trials for bone metastases. *Clin Oncol*, **24**(2), 112–24.

Goldstein N, Morrison RS (eds) (2012). *Evidence-Based Practice of Palliative Medicine*. Philadelphia, PA: Saunders.

Hanks G, Cherny NI, Christakis NA, Fallon M, Kassa S, Portenoy RK (eds) (2010). *Oxford Textbook of Palliative Medicine*. Oxford: Oxford University Press.

Hoskin PJ (2008). Opioids in context: relieving the pain of cancer. The role of comprehensive pain management. *Palliat Med*, **22**(4), 303–9.

Muller-Busch H, Andres I, Jehser T (2003). Sedation in palliative care – a critical analysis of 7 years experience. *BMC Palliat Care*, **2**(1), 2.

Zech DFK, Grond S, Lynch J, Hertel D, Lehmann KA (1995). Validation of the World Health Organization Guidelines for cancer pain relief. *J Pain*, **65**(1), 65–76.

Index

A

absolute alcohol, see alcohol block
adjuvants 25–7, 291–2
alcohol block 32, 33–4, 35, 37, 149, 158, 234
alcohol neuritis 37
algorithmic approach 139
alpha-2 adrenergic agonists 292
alternative therapies 300
amitriptyline 26, 27
anterior cingulotomy 258
anticonvulsants 26–7
antidepressants 26–7
aromatase inhibitors 54
Ascenda™ catheter 205

B

baclofen 26
balloon microcompression, Gasserian/trigeminal ganglion 243, 245–7
balloon tamp 177
benzodiazepines 26
bilateral cingulotomy 258
bilateral cordotomy 193
bisphosphonates 26, 55
bone pain 8
    adjuvants in hospice settings 292
    bisphosphonate therapy 26, 55
    external beam radiotherapy 56, 299
    incident pain 111–21
    intrathecal drug delivery 216
    radioisotopes 57, 299–300
bowel obstruction 292
brachial plexopathy 9
brainstem lesions 258
breakthrough pain 4, 5, 15
breast carcinoma 81
bupivacaine 201–2, 212, 215, 266, 296

C

cancer pain
    assessment 14, 286
    barriers to effective management 19
    causes 42
    clinical examination 15, 138
    definition 4
    epidemiology 5
    history 15, 138
    pathophysiology 7
    principles of effective management 16
    undertreatment 293
capsaicin 292
carbolic acid, see phenol block
case discussions
    bone pain 216
    breast carcinoma 81
    collaborative working 277
    diffuse lower body pain 90–7
    incident pain 114–20
    intrathecal pump 124–31
    lung carcinoma 83, 84
    mesothelioma and chest wall pain 71–6
    pelvic pain 63–5, 220
    perineal pain 218
    sacral and lumbar nerve root compression 222
    upper gastrointestinal pain from pancreatic cancer 102–7
    upper limb plexopathy pain 81–4
cauda equina compression 8
celecoxib 288
central sensitization 7
cervical cordotomy 181–94
    anatomical considerations 184
    bilateral 193
    complications 192
    contraindications 188
    efficacy 192
    historical background 183
    imaging 190
    indications 187
    myelogram 190–1
    patient positioning 189
    patient preparation 189
    postoperative care 192
    technique 189–92
    temperature perception 184, 192
cervical spine metastases 8

chemical neurolysis, see neurolysis
chemical neuromodulation 45, 255
chemotherapy 54
chest wall pain 8, 69–73, 265
chlorocresol 229, 231
chronic pain 4
clinical examination 15, 138
clonazepam 26, 27
clonidine 202, 212, 292
co-analgesics 25–7
codeine 20, 288–9
coeliac plexus neurolysis 150–9, 298
collaboration 273–82
comfort kit 287
commissural myelotomy 259
complementary therapies 300
complex cancer pain
    definition 4
    epidemiology 5
    pathophysiology 7
complex pain syndromes 8–9
COMT 22
consent 140
controlled sedation 301–2
cord compression 8
    post-vertebroplasty 175
    surgical decompression 253
cordotomy, surgical 259; see also cervical cordotomy
corticosteroids 25, 292
cryotherapy 32
CT-guided coeliac plexus block 155–6
CYP2D6 20

D

deep brain stimulation 254
denosumab 26, 55
dexamethasone 25
dextromethorphan 27
diamorphine 201
diazepam 26
diclofenac 20, 288
dihydrocodeine 20
documentation 138–9
dorsal root entry zone (DREZ) lesion 256, 259

double effect 295
drug treatment, see
    pharmacological
    management of pain
duloxetine 26, 27

E
e-kit 287
electrical neuromodulation
    45, 254–5
emergency kit 287
empowering patients 49
epidemiology of pain 5
epidural infusions 297
ethanol/ethyl alcohol, see
    alcohol block
ethical issues
    controlled sedation 302
    hospice settings 293–5
examination 15, 138
exemestane 54
external beam
    radiotherapy 56, 299

F
femoral nerve block 266
femoral neuralgia 266
fentanyl 24, 201, 212, 290
Flowonix catheter 206
Flowinix Prometra pump
    207
fluoroscopy-guided
    transcrural coeliac plexus
    block 154

G
gabapentin 26
gamma knife 256
ganglion impar block 163–5
Gasserian ganglion
    balloon microcompression
        243
    RF thermocoagulation
        243–4, 247
glioma surgery 252
glucocorticoids 292
glycerol block 36, 149

H
head and neck cancer,
    trigeminal interventions
    239–48
hip pain 266
history-taking 15, 138
hormones 54
hospice kit 287
hospice settings 285–303
    adjuvants 291–2
    analgesics 288–91
    comfort kit 287

complementary and
    alternative therapies 300
controlled sedation 301–2
ethical issues 293–5
interventional pain
    management 296–8
interventional pain
    specialist 85
opioid management 291
peripheral nerve
    blocks 264
radiation therapy 299–300
specific considerations for
    pain management 286
hydromorphone 201,
    212, 290
hyperbaric spinal
    neurolysis 232–3
hypobaric spinal
    neurolysis 234–5

I
ibuprofen 20, 288
incident pain 111–21
infection
    contraindication to
        intrathecal drugs 204
    post-vertebroplasty 175
inflammatory (nociceptive)
    pain 4, 14
informed consent 140
informed refusal 140
intercostal nerve block 265
intercostobrachial nerve
    block 265–6
interpleural block 298
interventional procedures
    algorithms 139
    assistance 142
    considerations during the
        procedure 143
    documentation 138–9
    history-taking 138
    hospice settings 296–8
    informed consent 140
    informed refusal 140
    investigations 138
    patient expectations 140
    patient positioning 142
    patient preparation 140–1
    physical examination 138
    postprocedure care 143
    radiology technicians 142
    surrogate
        decision-making 140
    timeout 142
    see also specific interventions
intracerebroventricular
    opioids 198
intractability 48–9
intrathecal drug
    delivery 197–224, 297
    ARCHIMEDES® pump 206

Ascenda™ catheter 205
battery-powered
    systems 207–8
bleeding diatheses 204
bone pain 216
bupivacaine 201–2,
    212, 215
bupivacaine, opioid
    and clonidine
    mixes 214–15
case discussion 123–32
clonidine 202, 212
complications 210
delivery systems 205–8
diagnosis 203
diamorphine 201
drug distribution 200
drugs 201–2
fentanyl 201, 212
fully implanted
    systems 205–8
gas-driven constant
    infusion system 206
granuloma 201, 211
hormone changes 211
hydromorphone 201, 212
hyperalgesia 211
implant procedure 210
infection 204
infusion regimens 212–15
ketamine 202
life expectancy 203
local anaesthetics 201–2
Medstream™ pump 205
methadone 202
morphine 201, 212
neurolytic agents 37
neurotoxic drugs 202
N'Vision® unit 208
opioids 201, 212–13
patient selection 203–4
patient therapy
    manager 208
pelvic pain 220
perineal pain 218
peripheral oedema 211
Polyanalgesic Consensus
    Conference
    recommendations
    199–200, 212
portacath systems 205
post-implant
    headache 211
pre-implantation MRI 203
psychiatric and
    psychological
    problems 204
sacral and lumbar
    nerve root
    compression 222
sulfentanil 212
Synchromed® II
    pump 207
test doses and trials 209

underuse 198, 255
Vygon ports 205
ziconotide 202, 203, 204, 212, 215
investigations 138

J

joint injections 296

K

ketamine 27, 91, 202
ketoprofen 20
ketorolac 288
knee pain 266
kyphoplasty 177, 296–7

L

lamotrigine 27
Leeds Assessment of Neuropathic Symptoms and Signs (LANSS) 14
lesions 45, 256–9
lidocaine 27, 292, 296
limbic lesions 258
LINAC-based systems 256
Liverpool model of collaboration 275–6
local anaesthetics 201–2, 296
lorazepam 302
lower body pain 89–99
lumbosacral plexopathy 9
lung cancer 8, 83, 84
luteinizing hormone-releasing hormone (LHRH) agonists 54

M

mandibular nerve 241
maxillary nerve 241
mesencephalotomy 258
mesothelioma 8, 69–77, 265
methadone 24–5, 27, 93, 202, 291
mexiletine 27
midazolam 302
midline myelotomy 259
morphine
  administration 21
  formulations 21
  hospice settings 289
  immediate release (IR) 21
  individual differences in response to 22
  intrathecal 201, 212
  modified (MR) 21
  side effects 23
  starting dose 21

switching to alternatives to 23
motor cortex stimulation 254–5
μ-opioid receptors 199
multidisciplinary teamworking 274

N

naproxen 288
nerve growth factors 7
nerve root compression 222
neural blockade 297–8
neuroablation (lesions) 45, 256–9
neurokinin-1 receptors 7
neurolysis 31–9, 267, 297–8
  alcohol block 32, 33–4, 35, 37, 149, 158, 234
  chlorocresol 229, 231
  coeliac plexus 150–9, 298
  ganglion impar 163–5
  glycerol block 36, 149
  interpleural 298
  intrathecal injection 37
  patient positioning 37, 38
  phenol block 32, 34, 35, 37, 149, 158, 229, 231
  selection of agent 37
  spinal 227–37
  superior hypogastric plexus 160–2, 298
neuromodulation 45, 254–5
neuropathic pain 4, 5, 14, 291
NMDA receptor antagonists 27
NMDA receptors 7
nociceptive pain 4, 14
non-opioid analgesics 20;
  see also specific drugs
non-steroidal anti-inflammatories (NSAIDs) 20, 288
nucleus caudalis DREZ lesions 259
N'Vision® unit 208

O

oncological management of pain 53–8
  bisphosphonates 55
  chemotherapy 54
  hormones 54
  radioisotopes 57
  radiotherapy 56
  targeted agents 54
ophthalmic nerve 241
opioid receptors 199
opioids
  addiction and abuse worries 294–5

common misconceptions 293–4
conversion factors 201
hospice settings 291
intracerebroventricular 198
intrathecal 201, 212–13
principle of double effect 295
switching to morphine alternatives 23
weak 20–1
see also morphine
outcomes 47
oxycodone 23, 289–90

P

pain, definition 4
palliation 42
palliative care, collaboration with pain medicine 273–82
pancreatic cancer 9, case discussion 102–7
coeliac plexus neurolysis 159
paracetamol 20, 288
paradoxical cerebral embolism 175
patient choice 49
patient expectations 140
pelvic pain 9, 61–7, 220
pentobarbital 302
percutaneous cervical cordotomy, see cervical cordotomy
percutaneous vertebroplasty, see vertebroplasty
perineal pain 218
periosteal pecking 265
peripheral nerve blocks 247, 263–8
peripheral sensitization 7
pharmacological management of pain 13–28
  adjuvants 25–7, 291–2
  adverse effects 23
  systemic approach to prescribing 20–1
  see also intrathecal drug delivery and specific drugs
phenobarbital 302
phenol block 32, 34, 35, 37, 149, 158, 229, 231
pituitary surgery 257–8
plasma-based RF ionization 178
polyanalgesic consensus conference recommendations 199–200, 212

portacath system 205
primary prescriber 19
principle of double
    effect 295
propofol 302
psychological distress 5
pulmonary embolism 175

R

radiofrequency techniques
    cervical cordotomy 191
    Gasserian/trigeminal
        ganglion 243–4, 247
    lesioning 256
    neurolysis 32
    tumour ablation
        combined with
        vertebroplasty 178
radioisotopes 57, 299–300
radiology technicians 142
radiopharmaceuticals 57,
    299–300
radiotherapy 56, 299–300
record-keeping 138–9
refusal of interventions 140
retrocrural coeliac plexus
    block 154

S

sacral and lumbar nerve root
    compression 222
secondary trigeminal
    neuralgia 240
sedation 301–2
sensory thalamotomy 258
shoulder pain 265
sodium valproate 27
soft tissue injections 296
somatic neural blocks 297
sorafenib 54
spinal cord compression 8
    post-vertebroplasty 175
    surgical
        decompression 253
spinal cord stimulation 254
spinal instability-related
    incident pain 113
spinal metastases 8
spinal neurolysis 227–37
spiritual pain 85
splanchnic block 154
stereotactic techniques 257
steroids 25, 292
structural outcome 47
subarachnoid neurolysis 37,
    235, 236
substance P 7
suffering 19, 85
sulfentanil 212

sunitinib 54
superior hypogastric
    plexus block/
    neurolysis 160–2, 298
suprascapular nerve
    block 265
surgical management of
    pain 41–50, 57, 251–60
    deposition of neurolytic
        agents 153
    intractability 48–9
    lesions 45, 256–9
    neuromodulation
        45, 254–5
    outcomes 47
    principles 44
    treatment of
        cause 44, 252
surrogate
    decision-making 140
sympathetic nerve
    blocks 148, 297;
    see also neurolysis
symptomatic outcome 47
Synchromed® II pump 207

T

tamoxifen 54
targeted agents 54
teamworking 274
TENS 254
thalamotomy 258
thiopental 302
thoracic spine
    metastases 8
timeout 142
tizanidine 292
topical anaesthetics 292
total pain 4, 85, 94
tramadol 289
transcranial magnetic
    stimulation 254–5
transcrural coeliac plexus
    block 153–4
transcutaneous electrical
    nerve stimulation 254
treatment of cause 44, 252
trigeminal ganglion 241
    RF/balloon
        microcompression
        243, 245–7
trigeminal
    interventions 239–48
trigeminal nerve 241
trigeminal
    neuralgia 240, 242
trigeminal neuropathy 240
trigger point injection 266
tumour-related trigeminal
    neuralgia 240

U

ultrasound-guided coeliac
    plexus block 157
ultrasound-guided ganglion
    impar block 165
ultrasound lesions 256
undertreatment of
    pain 293
upper gastrointestinal
    pain 101–8
upper limb plexopathy
    pain 79–87

V

venlafaxine 27
vertebral body
    metastases 8
vertebroplasty 167–79,
    296–7
    advantages 169
    bleeding risk 176
    cement allergy 176
    cement leakage 175
    collapse of adjacent
        vertebral body 175–6
    complications 175–6
    contraindications 172
    cord compression 175
    fracture risk 175
    historical background 168
    imaging 169–71
    infection risk 175
    mechanism of pain
        relief 169
    neurological deficits 175
    paradoxical cerebral
        embolism 175
    patient selection 169
    procedure 173–4
    pulmonary embolism
        175
    tumour ablative
        therapy 178
Vygon port 205

W

weak opioids 20–1
WHO analgesic ladder 48–9

X

Xofigo® 57

Z

ziconotide 199, 202, 203,
    204, 212, 215
zoledronic acid 26